THE JOURNEY BACK

ONE MAN'S FIGHT

ANNE PAPSODERO

PAGE PUBLISHING, INC.
Conneaut Lake, PA

First originally published by Page Publishing 2020

ISBN 978-1-64584-109-8 (pbk)
ISBN 978-1-64584-110-4 (digital)

Printed in the United States of America

CHAPTER ONE

My name is Anne, and I've heard people say that they have days that have changed their life forever. Well let me tell you; January 29, 2016, is a day that my life as I knew it changed forever. Let me backtrack a little bit for you. It was in 2008 when my husband, Michael, had his first attack of diverticulitis. We had gone to his brother's house one night for dinner during the summer that year. The music was on, and we were really enjoying ourselves. We were listening to classic rock, which we all loved. It was a warm night, and we were sitting in the screenhouse just enjoying life. After dinner his wife served a platter of fruit for dessert. Mike helped himself to the fruit. He was really enjoying it. He kept commenting on how good it was, especially the strawberries. I warned him to take it easy with the fruit. But of course, he didn't listen. He just kept right on eating them. We left some time around 11:00 p.m.

Later that night while we were sleeping, I woke up to hear him bellowing in pain. I rolled over and asked him what was wrong. He just kept screaming that his stomach hurt. I asked him if he could sit up and show me where the pain was. He couldn't even stand upright but said he was okay and would sleep it off. So I rolled over and went back to sleep. Finally he could no longer stand the pain and woke me up, and I took him to the hospital. On the way to hospital all he did was bellow that he was in pain. I was driving as fast as I could. As soon as we pulled up to the hospital I jumped out of the car and went screaming into the ER, saying that I needed a wheelchair for my husband. The security guard jumped to his feet and came running with the wheelchair. I didn't even park my car, I just left it where it was until I got him settled.

After a long night of tests, we were told that he has a condition called diverticulitis. We were told that he needed to be careful with what he ate, and he was given medication for the infection. Okay, I was familiar with this. My mom had surgery in 1976 for it. I remember it like it was yesterday, waiting for her to come home on that Christmas day. I was only six at the time, so I really didn't understand what had happened to her. I just know what my father had told me. I knew she was sick and at the hospital. I remember when she came home. I just stared at her. She looked like hell. She looked so weak and fragile, sitting in the gold chair in our dining room. She barely had the strength to lift her arm and wave at me as I was excitedly dancing in the dining room because I was so happy she was home. Hell, she didn't even have the strength to speak. Now thirty-two years later, I was experiencing it with my husband. And I knew the routine about what he should or shouldn't eat.

Over the next eight years, he was careful with what he ate. There were times when he had some discomfort from it. I always took him to the doctor or ER to be treated for it, and he was always given medicine to treat it. On the evening of January 25, 2016, when he started experiencing abdominal pain, I thought to myself, *Oh no, here we go again.* But this time was different. Something wasn't right to me. I took him to our local ER, which was County General, where they x-rayed him and said that yes, it is diverticulitis. We both asked them if they could give him something through his IV for his pain. They said no. They didn't have the proper pain meds to give him, so they sent him home with prescriptions and to follow-up with his primary care doctor at eleven forty-five that night.

Due to the late hour, there wasn't a pharmacy open for us to go to and get these filled, so we decided that we would go first thing in the morning. When we got home the girls were anxiously waiting for us. They asked if Mike was going to be okay. I said that of course he was. I told them that we had to go to the pharmacy in the morning to get his medication. They were happy to hear that and went to sleep. But sleep for me never happened that night as Mike was in excruciating pain. On top of Mike being sick, our dog was sick as well. It was around 3:00 a.m. when I heard Chase, our beagle, whimpering in his cage. Since I wasn't sleeping, I got up and went out to the living room to see what was wrong with him.

I looked at him and said, "*Now* you have to go?" So I let him out, and he made a beeline to the screenhouse. I opened the door and out he went. But would he go? *No!* He just kept whimpering. So I let him back in the house, and what does he do? He shits on my dining room rug! Great, just what I needed now was to clean up dog shit at three in the morning. I got out my bucket and filled it with soap and water and started cleaning my dining room rug. As I was doing this, I could see Mike crawling on his hands and knees to the bathroom. I called out to him and asked if he was okay.

He said, "Don't worry about me, just clean up the dog shit. It stinks!"

I said, "Oh yeah, you should be in here cleaning it. It's fucking horrible! It's like he had explosive diarrhea!"

Not only was Mike feeling pain from the diverticulitis he was also feeling pain from a herniated disk in his back. He said that it felt like a spear was going right through him. I asked him if he wanted me to massage his back. It always works for me. But he said no, he doesn't like massages. He hurt his back in October when he was helping his brother move. He moved a workbench and twisted the wrong way and herniated a disk on his lower left side of his back. Occasionally he would have some pain from it, but he always managed it.

Since it was late at night, I didn't want to call my mother-in law Kathy. She also lived an hour away. I also didn't want to leave my girls home alone at that late hour, but I was torn about making that decision. Mike said that he just needed some sleep and that he would be fine. But at six thirty the next morning, I decided that we could wait no longer. So I called Kathy and told her that she needed to come to my house that afternoon after work to stay with my girls. Kathy is a substitute teacher at Sunny Elementary School in Kissimmee. I told her what was going on and where I was going.

As I drove to the hospital, I was thinking well that he might be admitted for a day or two then spend two days at home recovering and then go back to work. I couldn't have been more wrong. As I suspected he was admitted to the hospital. While waiting with Mike in the triage area, he was given some medicine through his IV for his pain and they were treating the infection as well. I breathed a sigh of relief and was thanking God that he was feeling somewhat better and not in as much pain anymore. I made the usual phone calls to our families to let them know what was going on and told them he was being admitted to the hospital. He finally got a room at four that afternoon. Once we were in his room, I called Kathy and asked her to please bring me clothes as I was going to be spending the night with Mike. She said that she would and bring my daughters, eighteen-year-old Elizabeth and eleven-year-old Alexandra, up to see Mike. You see my oldest daughter, Danielle, who was twenty-one at the time, had moved back home to New York. But I was in constant communication with her, letting her know what was going on with Mike.

By the morning of January 27, Mike was feeling somewhat better, but they refused to feed him. What? How do you refuse to feed a patient but at the same time pump him with medication? It didn't make any sense to me, but I thought, *Hey, the doctors know what they are doing right?* He was so hungry, and I thought that this isn't right, he needed some food in his system. He was hallucinating and seeing a giant M&M clock on the wall. He kept saying, "I want M&Ms. That's all I want. I'm so hungry. Why won't they feed me?"

My heart was breaking, and I couldn't stand to see him like this. So I marched right out to the nurses' station and said, "Feed my husband."

The nurses looked startled because I am four feet eleven inches tall and here I was screaming at them to bring Mike some food. So they contacted the doctor and finally he could eat. He started slowly with clear liquids, but hey, he was eating. Dr. Anjali came in and spoke with us about having the surgery. He informed us that Mike would have a colostomy bag for six months but that it would be temporary and eventually removed. We just looked at each other. I knew inside that Mike was terrified.

He turned to me and said, "If I wake up from this surgery with a bag, I'm jumping out that fucking window! Whatever you do, don't let that bald motherfucker touch me!"

I told him that I wouldn't. Later that day another surgeon by the name of Dr. Cruz came to his room and spoke with Mike about operating on his back as well. Not only did they want to perform a bowel resection but they wanted to operate on his back too. He had called me on the phone to tell me this. My head was spinning at this point. I thought, *How can they do two operations at once? Is that even possible?*

All day doctors were coming and going, checking on Mike. At some point another surgeon named Alex Lopez came to check on my husband and discuss the same surgery with him. He called me and asked my opinion. I asked him if he told Dr. Alex Lopez what Dr. Anjali had told him about the colostomy bag. He said that he had and that's what Dr. Lopez wanted to talk to both of us about. Mike was informed that they would not be doing the back surgery as it would have been too much for him to handle all at once. On the morning of January 28, I did just that, both Mike and I spoke with Dr. Lopez. I expressed my concerns with the surgery. I informed him again about what Dr. Anjali had told us, and he said that Dr. Anjali was talking out of his ass and not to pay attention to what he was saying. Feeling apprehensive I agreed. He told me that they were going to give Mike something called "GoLYTELY" to clean out his intestines. I asked if this was necessary. He said yes. What could I do? He was the doctor and he knew what was best, right?

Still when I left the hospital, I couldn't help but have an uneasy feeling about it. I tried to push those feelings away, but I just couldn't. As I headed to work that afternoon, my emotions were running high. I told Mike that I would be back that night to stay with him. I called him on my fifteen-minute break, and he said that he was feeling nervous about the surgery. I tried to assure him that everything would be okay. He wasn't convinced. My break was ending, and I told him that I loved him and that I would see him later.

He then said to me, "Well time for me to set up a table for my shit fest."

I laughed and said, "What?"

He said, "I'm preparing myself to get ready and drink that shit to clean out my intestines."

I told him not to forget that he could mix it with Gatorade or water and to make sure the nurse knew too. He said that he would do that. I left work at 9:40 p.m. that night. I called Mike from my car, and he did not sound well at all. I asked him what was wrong. He told me that his belly was all distended and that he couldn't shit and he couldn't puke. What the hell? This doesn't sound right at all. I told him that I was on my way. He said that his father and Suzy were going too. I rushed to the hospital as fast as I could. When I arrived, my father-in-law, Tom, and his wife, Suzy, were already there taking care of Mike. Mike was sitting at the edge of his bed and vomiting uncontrollably into a basin. His father had put cold towels around his neck and wrapped him in a blanket to keep him warm. I told him to immediately stop drinking the GoLYTELY.

Once again, I marched out to nurses' station and demanded that they call the doctor. The nurse on duty, Nancy, came in and I said to her, "Mike is not going to finish the rest of the GoLYTELY. You need to contact the doctor and find another way to prep him for the surgery."

She came back a few minutes later and said that Dr. Anjali said to administer an enema. Again what could I do? Even though Mike was so sick, he still had a sense of humor. He turned around and said, "An *enema*! I've never taken it in the ass before."

His father said, "Well guess what you are now, buddy, so get ready."

So the enema was given to Mike. By this time Tom and Suzy were getting ready to leave and told me to call them if I needed anything.

I changed my clothes, got my PJS on, and laid on the pullout chair next to Mike's bed. Well as you can imagine, sleep never came. I was up all night with Mike because once again he was in excruciating pain. The nurse, Nancy, did nothing. I begged her to give Mike something for his pain. She finally gave him something, but it didn't help. As I tried to sleep, all night, Mike kept saying to me that he was going to die on the table. I kept assuring him that he wouldn't, but I myself wasn't sure. At 7:00 a.m., Kathy was there. I asked why she was there. She said that she was worried. Worried was an understatement. They came in and got Mike. We followed him down to the surgical pre-op area. As I stood there waiting for them to wheel him back to surgery, I had this overwhelming feeling that I would never see him alive again.

At one point he asked for our oldest daughter, Danielle. He kept asking me if she was coming. I told him that she lived in New York now and that she wouldn't be coming. Oh, but she would be there, he just wouldn't be seeing her. I was running on no sleep, and my emotions were on overload. But once again I put my faith in the doctors that everything would be okay. I was crying uncontrollably. Kathy kept telling me not to because it would upset Mike. What? Why should I stop crying? This was my husband, the father of my three daughters; how was I supposed to feel? Kathy left, and I was alone with my thoughts. I was pacing like an expectant father would, anticipating the arrival of a child.

When they came and got Mike, Dr. Lopez looked at Mike and then looked at me and said, "What the hell happened to him?"

I explained the events from the night before. He advised the nurse to give him something for the pain. They asked him all the usual questions: his name, date of birth, why he was there, and who the surgeon was. He answered all of them correctly too. As far as the doctor was concerned there was no reason to worry. Believe me I was worried. I leaned over and kissed him and told him that I loved him and that I would see him later. I was mentally and physically exhausted at this point. I just wanted to go home and sleep. I walked as far as they would let me go and stopped by the elevator. Mike was reaching for me, and I reached out to him and said I love you. As I stepped on the elevator, I said a little prayer. I prayed all the way home.

CHAPTER TWO

When I got home, I showered and went to sleep. I was awoken some time later by the sound of my daughter Elizabeth's voice saying, "Mom, your cell phone is ringing."

I immediately jumped up, grabbed it to see who had called me. It was the hospital. I looked at the time, and it was 11:30 a.m. I frantically tried calling them back but was unable to reach the surgeon. Little did I know that a simple act such as returning a phone call would shatter my life as I knew it. So I grabbed my car keys and said to Elizabeth, "Let's go now."

Still trying to call the hospital as I was driving, they called me. I pulled over, and the surgeon, Dr. Lopez, was telling me that the surgery went well, *but* he found something. *Oh, shit,* I thought. What did he find? The first thing that came to mind was colon cancer. Mike had three polyps removed in 2013. I asked him what it was. He said that Mike was filled with pus. I nearly dropped my phone but kept my composure.

I said, "What?"

Again he said that he was filled with pus.

"How?" I asked.

He said that Mike had an abscess that somehow went undetected and ruptured. He told me that he was able to remove all the pus, *but* Mike was sick, he was very sick. I was in such a state of shock and had no idea just how sick Mike was. He told me that Mike would be in the ICU for a few days and should be able to go home at the end of the week. I thought, *Okay that doesn't sound too bad.* He told me the that the ICU was located on the second floor of the hospital.

Not knowing what I was going to encounter, I rushed to the hospital as fast as I could. I went to the family waiting area for surgical patients in the ICU. I was shaking. I asked about Mike because I didn't see his name on the board that they had. They told me that he was in recovery and that Dr. Lopez would be with me shortly. Still shaking I sat down with Elizabeth and began to pray. I even went on my Facebook page and asked everyone near and far to please pray for my sick husband. Finally, after what seemed like an eternity, someone said my name. I looked up and they said, "Come with me."

I took my daughter's hand and followed this person. I was greeted by the surgeon, Dr. Lopez. He told me again that Mike was okay and that he was in recovery but that he would be in the ICU for a few days. He again told me that there was an abscess that had ruptured and that's where the pus came from. He also said that the pus was leaking in to Mike's body all night. I now had a better understanding of the abdominal pain that Mike was having the night before.

I asked him, "How was this not seen on any of the MRIs that were done?"

He just looked at me and shrugged his shoulders. He just didn't know. He then told me to go back to the waiting room and that I would be able to see Mike shortly. What he didn't tell me at the time was as I was headed back to the waiting room; he had been paged by the recovery room and was told, "Hey, your patient is coding." Which basically means that at that very moment, Mike was dying.

He replied to the recovery nurse, "What the fuck are you talking about? I just told his wife that he was going to be fine. Work on him now! I'm on my way to the recovery room."

After another agonizing wait, I heard someone call my name and say, "You can go see your husband now. He's in room 2210."

Not knowing what to expect, I took my daughter's hand and rushed to his room where I was stopped and told that I couldn't go in. The curtain was pulled all the way over which obstructed my view. All I could see was silhouettes of doctors rushing around working on Mike. I kept trying to see around the curtain, but I couldn't. I was ushered in to the ICU waiting room where I waited for Mike's family to arrive. His mother, Kathy, his brother, Tom, and his father, Tom, all arrived about the same time.

A nurse then peeked her head in and said, "I'm looking for the wife."

I said that's me, raising my hand ever so slowly. She said that I had a phone call. A phone call? Who the hell could possibly be calling me here? I followed the nurse to where the phone was, and I picked up the phone and said, "Hello?"

The voice on the other end was my father Tom's wife, Patty. She said, "Hi, honey. How are you? Dad wants to talk to you."

I thought to myself, *Of all the people to track me down, it would be him to find me like a bloodhound.* He got on the phone and peppered me with questions about Mike's condition. He asked if I wanted him to come on Saturday. I said yes. I also wished him a happy birthday since it was the same day. You see my mom, Camille, was scheduled for hip replacement surgery that Monday and was unable to make the trip from Port Charlotte, Florida, as it was a three-hour car ride for her.

I hung up the phone and returned to the waiting room. You might be a little confused with the family situation. You see both our parents are divorced and have significant others except for Kathy. I explained to them that my dad had called. They asked if he was coming; I told them that he would be there on Saturday. He lives in Fort Pierce, Florida, which is about 1.5 hours away.

CHAPTER THREE

The nurse came in again, and we were then ushered into an even smaller waiting room. As we waited an ICU doctor named Dr. Neel came in and sat down and started peppering me with all these medical terms. He told me that he worked on Mike for forty minutes and that Mike was now in a medically induced coma due to the sepsis. Sepsis? What the hell is that? He then informed me that Mike had been oxygen deprived and he didn't know for how long. He also told me that Mike had a condition called ARDS and that 30 percent of patients with this condition don't make it. ARDS is short for Adult Respiratory Distress Syndrome. What? None of this made any sense to me. Mike was a healthy man before this. I needed to get out of this room before I lost it. I stood up, and I threw my glasses across the room and nearly collapsed, but thankfully Elizabeth caught me.

After that it's all blur. I remembered hearing the doctor's voice, but what he was saying, I didn't know. I remembered speaking to Danielle and telling her what was happening, but everything was fuzzy. I tried the best I could to explain everything. Danielle called me back in tears and said that she would be in Florida by ten the next morning. I remembered speaking to my cousin, Caroline. I remembered saying to her that Mike couldn't die because he had to see my girls get married. Caroline tried to comfort me and said "Don't worry Mike is strong. He'll make it through this, I promise."

As we all sat there in shock, all I could think of was Alexandra being home by herself and not knowing what the hell was going on. At the time I didn't know that Danielle had called and spoke to Alexandra and told her she was coming down the next day. She had no idea what was happening, but she soon would. At the same time,

I wanted to see Mike, but I wasn't sure I could handle seeing him. So I told everyone that I needed to go home to be with Alexandra.

They kept saying to me, "Don't you want to see Mike?"

I said, "Of course, I do, but I have an eleven-year-old daughter who has no idea what the hell is going on, and I need to be home for her."

Kathy turned and said, "Okay, everybody, calm down. She needs to be home for Alex. That little girl has no idea what the hell is going on and needs her mom. If anything she can come back later, if she feels up to it. Right now she is running on no sleep and hasn't eaten anything at all today." We then got up and left.

Elizabeth and I got in my car, and Kathy followed behind.

While I was driving home, I was numbed and trying to process the day's events. Also I was trying to find the right words to tell Alexandra what has happened to her dad. As I was driving home, my cell phone rang, and it was my mom. She asked me how I was doing. I explained to her that I myself was still trying to process what happened.

She started crying and said to me, "How could this happen? He's a young, healthy man."

Both Elizabeth and I started to cry again. Through tears I told her that I was still trying to understand it myself. I also told her that I spoke to my dad and that he was coming up the next day. She was glad that he would be there.

As I pulled up to my apartment, I could see Alexandra happily walking our dog Chase. She skipped happily over to my car window and said, "Hi, Mommy! How's Daddy?" I guess she must've seen the look on my face because the next words out of her mouth were "Did he die?"

I just looked at her and said, "Let's go in the house." I got her in the house, sat her down at the kitchen table, and explained everything to her.

Her eyes were wide as saucers, and she just broke down crying. My heart was breaking. My only saving grace was that Danielle would be here in the morning, and I couldn't wait. It might sound selfish, but with Danielle around, life is a little easier. The girls really look up to her and love having her around. Poor Elizabeth was with me all day and was very stressed, and I didn't know if she would be able to go up to the hospital tomorrow. That little girl is tougher than she looked. So I asked Kathy if she would stay with me.

"Absolutely," she said. But she needed to go home and get clothes. So she took Alexandra with her. I asked her if she would pick up dinner for us as we had not eaten all day. She asked, "Is McDonald's okay?"

I said yes. At this point I would've settled for anything. I knew she would be gone for at least two hours, so I decided to take a shower. As I stood there with the water running on me, I just lost it. I just couldn't understand why this was happening to us. This is something that you would see in a movie, not real life. Not my life. The thought of me being a widow at forty-five scared the shit out of me. I just pushed that thought right out of my head. After my shower I put my pajamas on and just collapsed in a heap on my bed. I was mentally, emotionally, and physically exhausted. I just needed a good night's sleep. Kathy returned sometime later with dinner.

While we were eating, Suzy called and told me that I needed to go to the hospital and wanted to know why I didn't stay to see Mike. I said to her, "Suzy, I have another daughter that needed me. I don't need this guilt right now. I am exhausted beyond words and need a good night's sleep. I am also trying to eat! I will be there in the morning as soon as Danielle gets here."

She really didn't say much and just said okay, and we hung up. We did the best we could to eat. I finally went to bed at around nine thirty that night. I just wanted to wake up from this nightmare.

CHAPTER FOUR

At six thirty the next morning, I heard Kathy scurrying around the kitchen. She called out to me and said that Mike had shown a slight improvement overnight. She told me that she was going up to the hospital. I admit I was a little happy, but I knew that anything could happen. I told her that I would be there once Danielle got here.

I got up at around eight thirty that morning, and the smell of coffee was all through the house. I wasn't hungry, but a nice cup of coffee sounded good. I was still in shock from everything that happened. I got dressed and just sat on the couch and drank my coffee. At 10:00 a.m. there was a knock on the door. It was Danielle. I was elated. The girls were happy and so was the dog. Her friend, Michelle, had picked her up from the airport. I couldn't thank her enough. I was in no shape to drive, so I just handed Danielle my car keys. I asked Elizabeth if she wanted to come and she said no. I couldn't blame her. I knew she needed time to just digest what had just happened. She asked me if I was mad. How could I be? This little girl was my rock yesterday and witnessed a hell of a lot. I told her that I loved her and that I would text her at some point during the day. So Danielle, myself, Michelle, and Alex all piled in my car and off we went to the hospital.

Once at the hospital (County General), I had no idea what to expect. I checked in at the desk where they took a lovely picture of me and the girls too. As I rode the elevator to the ICU floor, I didn't know what I would be walking into. I got off the elevator and headed straight for Mike's room. I walked down the hall toward his room with Alexandra holding my hand and my heart pounding in my chest.

I saw Kathy coming out of his room with her arms outstretched and said to me, "Why? Why?"

She was referring to why I brought Alexandra up to the hospital. I simply said that it's her father and she wanted to see him. Tensions were high, but I was not in the mood for any arguments. So I slowly walked into to his room, and what I saw nearly took my breath away. There was Mike hooked up to all these machines with IVs everywhere. There was a machine breathing for him. All I heard were the sounds these machines were making. It's a sound that I will never forget and hopefully never have to hear again. I guess my knees were getting weak because the next thing I knew, a nurse was pushing a chair under me, and I just went down into it. I was crying and holding Mike's hand and telling him that I loved him and that I would be right here by his side. Out of the corner of my eye, I saw Danielle. She was leaning on Kathy and crying.

Alexandra was holding Mike's hand and said, "My poor Daddy. My poor, poor Daddy." I looked at her and saw the tears streaming down her face and falling onto the sheets. I just sat there and stared at him.

I must've been sitting there for God knows how long because the next thing I knew, Danielle was tapping me on the shoulder, telling me my dad was there. I got up and turned and saw him and Patty out in the hall. I went out there and stood next to him, waiting for him to say something to me, but I guess he didn't recognize me with my new glasses on because he looked around and said, "Where the hell is Anne?"

I tapped him and said that I'm right here, and at the same time Patty said the same thing to him. He then looked at me and said, "Oh my god." We both chuckled and then he hugged me and asked me how I was doing. I said that I'm here. He just stared at Mike in disbelief. You see Mike and him never had the greatest relationship. It had been tumultuous at times. My dad had his own health issues. He had undergone quadruple bypass surgery in 2015. But he was here for me, and I was extremely thankful for that. He and Patty went to the ICU waiting room to sit down for a while. I sat with Mike a little while longer, just listening to the machine that was pumping the fluid out of his lungs. I watched his chest go up and down as it pumped the fluid out. I felt like I was in a movie watching someone else's life. I was so numb I didn't know what to feel. I kept thinking, *Is this real or am I dreaming?*

I needed a break but at the same time felt guilty for leaving him alone. So I went to the ICU waiting room to catch my breath. While sitting there I remembered seeing on TV that coma patients can hear you even though they are unconscious. I even brought up some pictures, but the nurse said I wasn't allowed to display them. So after taking a little break, I went back to sit with Mike and started talking to him. I asked the nurse if I could put the TV on. She said that I could. I put his favorite channel on. The History channel. He loved to watch *Modern Marvels*. That wasn't on, so I just left what was on at the time on. I sat there, held his hand, and rubbed it and told him that he was going to be okay. I didn't even know if that was true myself. I needed to stay positive.

I eventually called my job and told them that I wouldn't be in the whole week due to Mike's condition. I spoke with my manager, Chris, and he said not to worry, that he would take me off the schedule and to call him when I was ready to come back. I thanked him, and he said that's not a problem. I went back and forth to the waiting room for a while. My dad had taken my girls downstairs to the cafeteria for some lunch to keep their minds off what was going on. Which I was truly thankful for.

It was somewhere between four thirty and five when Kathy said that she was going back to my house. She told me that she was going to pick up some fried chicken at Publix Supermarket. I thought, *Wow, that sounded good, considering I hadn't eaten at all that day.* I think I had a cup of coffee that morning. I asked my dad if he and Patty wanted to come to my house for dinner. He said that he was feeling tired and was going to head home. I couldn't blame him. I hugged him and thanked him for coming, and I told him that I would keep him posted about Mike's condition. I eventually went home at seven. I was exhausted and drained from everything.

CHAPTER FIVE

Once we got home all I wanted was a nice, hot shower and my bed. Now I'm not the most religious person around, but as I was showering, I swear I could hear Mike talking to me. I could hear him saying to me, "I can't do this anymore. I'm tired of fighting this. I'm not strong enough. You'll be fine without me. You're a strong person, you can handle it."

I spun around in the tub because I was freaked out. I just started talking out loud. I said, "Don't you dare leave me! You are strong enough to fight this! So fight it, damn it! Don't you know everyone is praying for you? Danielle flew in to see you!"

I really felt like I was losing my mind just standing there naked and wet in my shower and talking. I got out of the shower and got my pajamas on and laid on my bed to rest. I tried to call my cousin, Caroline, because I needed someone to talk to about what just happened while I was showering. I couldn't reach her, so I just sat on the couch and watched TV. I tried to eat, but it wasn't working. My dad had told me all day that I needed to eat and rest. I didn't have the energy to eat. With whatever energy I did have, I went on Facebook and group messaged all of Mike's friends and told them what was going on. Within minutes I was receiving phone calls from them. They were in shock. They wanted to know how this could have happened. They were asking if there was anything that they could do. I just told them to pray. That's all I wanted anyone to do, just pray.

I explained to them what had happened. I was attempting to eat something when Kathy told me that she was going back up to the hospital. I said to her, "Now? At this late hour? What for?" She told me that she wanted to. What could I do? I wasn't going to argue with her, after all that's her son. You see Mike's brother, Tom, had been through a lot with his diabetes. But that's another story altogether. Mike was always the rock in the family, and now here he was fighting for his life.

So out the door she went. Little did I know that Caroline would be coming back with her. What I didn't know at the time was that Caroline was up at the hospital visiting Mike. She was telling him that he needed to wake up and get better because we had a vacation planned for that summer. She was yelling at him and crying at the same time. She loved Mike like a brother, and it was very hard for her to see him like that. About an hour later, Caroline called me, and as I was talking to her, there was a knock at my door. I opened the door and there staring back at me was Caroline. I just hugged her and cried. I now knew why Kathy said that she had to go back to the hospital. I spent some time with Caroline. She couldn't stay very long, but the few minutes she was there was nice. She was only in town for the weekend with Jack and the boys. They were looking at colleges in Tampa for her son, Christopher. They were leaving in the morning. By this time it was ten thirty, and I needed to go to sleep. We said our goodbyes, and I promised her that I would keep her up-to-date on Mike's condition.

CHAPTER SIX

On Sunday mornings Mike would make pancakes for breakfast. But this Sunday morning, no one was in the mood for pancakes. Even though Elizabeth said that she would make them, it just wasn't the same without Mike. So at around twelve thirty, we all headed up to the hospital. To my surprise, when we got to Mike's room, his best friend, Mike, and his wife, Maria, were there. They lived in Fort Lauderdale. I was so happy to see them. They were very concerned for me. Maria hugged me, and I just started bawling. It was hard for them to see Mike like this. Hell, it was hard for me to see Mike like this! What Mike didn't tell me at the time was that right before I got there, Mike's heart rate started to drop dramatically while he was in the room with him. While standing there, he said doctors and nurses were rushing around Mike to stabilize him. He thought to himself, *Oh my God, I am going to watch my best friend die right in front of me.* He started to cry because he couldn't handle it. Thankfully they were able to stabilize him.

We went to the ICU waiting room and sat down and talked for a bit. You see I had been friends with all of Mike's friends for the last twenty-seven years, and we were like a little family. They were all at our wedding, and they were all there when each of the girls were born. I hosted many Sunday afternoon football parties with them. I loved having them around. We had so much fun and lots of laughs over the years. So it was nice to have Mike and Maria there. We talked a lot about the old days and all the fun we had. That made me feel a little bit better. As we were sitting there talking about the old days, Mike mentioned to me that Mikes godparents had come up to visit him. I looked at him with a very perplexed look on my face. "What?" I said. He said that it was an older couple that was up there.

I asked him how he knew that. He said that he had a conversation with them. I explained that his godparents live in NY and that they weren't married to each other. He again said, "Well that's who they said they were." To this day, I have no idea who this mystery couple was.

I went back to Mike's room to sit with him some more and talk to the nurse who was taking care of him. The nurse said that he was improving slowly. But only time will tell at this point. All we could do now was just wait and see what happens. While I was sitting with Mike, I was feeling very overwhelmed, and I just needed to splash some water on my face. So I went to the bathroom that was in his hospital room, and I just stood there and stared at my reflection in the mirror. As I looked at myself, I thought, *Wow, have I aged.* The stress was written all over my face. My hair was graying, my eyes were sunken in, and I was very pale. I looked terrible. But I didn't care. My main concern was Mike. So I splashed water on my face and went back to sit with Mike.

I was just sitting there, staring at him and holding his hand and watching the machine breathe for him. I just couldn't leave him alone. I felt an enormous amount of guilt if I went into the waiting room for a break. While I was sitting there, Dr. Lopez came in to check on Mike. He was checking his IV bags, and as he was doing this, he picked up the drain that was in Mike's incision and said very casually, "Oh, he has e-coli."

I jumped up out of my chair and said, "*What*! That's the last thing he needs right now! How serious is it?"

He said, "Ah, he'll be fine."

I'm thinking to myself, *I'm glad you think he's going to be fine.* He told me that his condition was improving slowly and not to lose hope. He then left, and I sat back down again. I don't know how long I was sitting there when Danielle came in and tapped me on my shoulder and said, "C'mon, you need a break. You need to eat something. This isn't healthy for you to constantly sit here." She couldn't have been more right. She took me by my arm and said, "Let's go downstairs and get something to eat. Leave your purse. I'll pay."

So down we went. I was just starting to relax and enjoy some food when Danielle's cell phone rang. It was Kathy. She was screaming into the phone, "Where's Mommy? I need to talk to her." Danielle handed me the phone.

I grabbed the phone and said, "What's the matter? What happened?"

She said, "You need to get back up here. You need to sign some papers."

Well so much for getting something to eat. Instead of telling the nurse that I went to get something to eat and that I would sign the papers when I came back up, she called Danielle in a panic. So I went back upstairs and found the nurse. She informed me that I was to sign these forms stating that I was the only one to make any medical decisions for Mike according to the state of Florida. So without any hesitation, I signed them. Well as you can imagine, that didn't go over well with his family. They felt that they should be the ones making all the medical decisions for Mike. But you know what? I really didn't give a shit what anyone thought. Mike is my husband and the father of my children. I was doing everything on my own. No one was helping me. No one was offering to help me with any of the bills. Yes, Kathy was staying with me, but she wasn't paying anything for me. Don't get me wrong, I truly appreciated that she was staying with us, but not once did she offer to even pay any of my bills. I'm not saying that I expected her to do it, but at least make the offer. For God's sake I had to apply for food stamps so I could put food on the table for my kids! I was the only one working. I also had to file for Mike's short-term disability benefits and try to get Social Security disability benefits as well. This was all so overwhelming for me, but I had to do it. After all I didn't have much of a choice.

I was talking to the nurse about Mike's condition and how he was doing. Again she said that it would be a slow process and that I had to take it day by day. She informed me that the doctors were concerned that Mike's kidneys weren't functioning properly due to his poor urine output. She said that he was going to have hemodialysis. I took a deep breath and thought, *Just one more hurdle that we must overcome.* As if we hadn't had enough to overcome in our married life.

Starting with the birth of Danielle, that was a nightmare. I had to have an emergency C-section with her, and I honestly thought that I would never be able to have any more kids after her. My placenta started to separate from my uterus, and I was hemorrhaging, and they couldn't track her heartbeat on the fetal monitor. Talk about scary? They wouldn't even let Mike in the room when they delivered her. They had the NICU team in the delivery room waiting for her to be born.

When she was finally born, she wasn't breathing, and they couldn't find her heartbeat. It was a living hell, much like what I am going through right now. Now twenty-one years later, she was my rock that I was leaning on right now along with Elizabeth and Alexandra. So I continued to talk to the nurse regarding Mike's condition. I asked her when the dialysis might start. She said that was up to the doctor. I asked when the doctor would be there, and she said in the morning. I just looked at Kathy and started to cry.

She reached out and hugged me and said, "I think it's time we all go home. It's been a very long day."

Once again I was consumed with guilt because I was leaving Mike alone. The nurse assured me that if anything were to happen, they would call me. I made sure that the phone number that they had was correct. I went into Mike's room and kissed him on the far head, told him I loved him and that I would see him tomorrow. We all headed to the elevator to go home. I just wanted to go to sleep and be alone.

CHAPTER SEVEN

When we got home, I took a shower and just collapsed on my bed. I just laid there and stared at the ceiling. My cell phone was on my night table and that's where it would stay until Mike was home. Though I was extremely tired, I just couldn't sleep. My thoughts were focused on Mike. I also was focused on how I was going to pay my bills in the coming months. I mean what was I going to do? My car needed a tire, and I didn't have the money to get one. Danielle said that she would take my car to Sam's Club and get one during the week for me. We both used to work there, and everyone there was praying for us as well. She also said that she would go to Publix and get some groceries for us. Will this ever end? I wondered when life would be back to normal.

The next day, which I believe was Monday, when I got up to the hospital, I saw that Mike had already started hemodialysis. I asked the nurse that was taking care of him how long he would have to be on dialysis. She said that as of right now it was going to be continuous until his urine output was enough. I just kept shaking my head because honestly, I didn't understand anything. I mean I knew what dialysis was because my brother-in-law used to have it done, but that was for his diabetes.

I said to the nurse, "He's not diabetic, so why does he have to have this done?"

She replied, "It's to jump-start his kidneys so that he would have a better urine output."

She also informed me that it was also to keep his kidneys functioning. I just stood there, too numb to move. Was I hearing her right? Was she telling me that his kidneys were failing? So I asked her if they were, and she said no, that they want to make sure that they wouldn't. I breathed a little sigh of relief. Once again I put my faith in the fact that the doctors knew better than I did. She also told me that Mike had developed bilateral pneumonia. *Oh great, more problems for him.* I just stood there in shock. Was there anything else that could possibly happen to him? The day hadn't started out all that great to begin with.

Danielle and Elizabeth had gone to pick up Alexandra early from school. Elizabeth went in since I was up at the hospital. When she went to sign her out, Janet, who is the desk clerk, said to her, "Can't she wait until the end of the day to see her father?" Now Elizabeth, who is very timid and shy, didn't say anything to her. That night, as we were all getting ready for bed, Elizabeth mentioned the incident.

Well Danielle came flying out of the bathroom and around the corner into the living room and said, "*What! Why didn't you tell me?*"

Elizabeth shrugged her shoulders and said, "I don't know."

Danielle was livid. "If this bitch thinks she's gonna get away with this, she's wrong."

I had gotten notes from the hospital saying that Mike was in a coma because Danielle needed them for work. My plan was to keep Alexandra home on Thursday so she could spend time with Mike; she really wasn't able to concentrate on school anyway, so I figured why not keep her home.

So on Thursday the four of us got ready to go to the hospital. Danielle, who was still pissed about what happened on Monday, was pacing like a caged animal, talking out loud about what she was going to say to Janet. We got in my car and headed for the school. We made Alex duck down in the car so no one would be able to see her. We parked the car. Danielle and I got out and headed for the office. I told her to relax and not to lose her cool. We entered the office and walked straight up to the desk where Janet was sitting.

This bitch lifted her head up, and in the worst southern drawl I ever heard said, "Can I help y'all?"

Danielle thrust the note in her hand toward her and told her who we are. She told Janet, "This is a note for my sister for missing school and being picked up early to go see my dad in the hospital.

You see my dad is in a coma, and we don't know what his outcome will be. So to answer your stupid question from the other day, *no*, she can't wait until the end of the day to see her dad. We don't know if he'll be alive or dead by the end of the day!"

Janet's face turned about six shades of red. She dropped her head and had nothing to say. She looked at us and said, "I am so sorry. I had no idea what was going on."

Danielle looked at her dead in the eye and said, *"Exactly*! So don't just sit there and assume you do!"

We turned and left, not giving her any opportunity to respond. It was great. Danielle was exactly like her father would've been had it been any other situation. She really was a daddy's girl at heart. When I got up to the hospital, I noticed another doctor sitting outside Mike's room going over his records. His name was Dr. Gomez, the head of nephrology, and he was livid. I just stood there and listened to the conversation he was having with the nurse. I heard him say things like "Who wanted him on continuous dialysis?" To which the nurse replied, "Dr. Navin." He's a kidney doctor that Tom had gone to.

He then said, "Well get him off it now! Can't you see its drying him out?"

I entered his room and took one look at Mike, and sure enough his skin looked like that of an alligator. I spoke to this new doctor, and he informed me that Mike would be on dialysis only when he needed it and that he should've never been put on continuous dialysis in the first place. He then told me that my brother-in-law, Tom, was the one who spoke to Dr. Navin regarding putting Mike on continuous dialysis.

Well that was the straw that broke the camel's back. I had just about enough of his brother interfering with Mike's care. I mean there were days when Tom would come up and play music for Mike. He would play AC/DC for him, which one of his favorite bands to listen to, and I appreciated that but don't think you can interfere with his health care. Next my father-in-law insisted that his wife's infectious disease doctor, Dr. Anika, should see Mike because he didn't like the one that was assigned to Mike. Now this? I'm his wife, damn it! I'll be the one making decisions for his care and no one else! I informed the male nurse on duty that no one is to discuss Mike's condition with anyone but me. He said that he would do that. Well as you can imagine, that did not go over well with his family. They insisted that they be kept in the loop when it came to his medical care. I didn't give a damn on what they thought. As far as I was concerned, they were on a need-to-know basis. When they needed to know something, I would be the one to tell them until then they were not going to be informed of anything.

That night when Kathy got home, she took me by the hand into my room and insisted that I put Mike's father on the paper that I signed on Sunday. I told her no, that by law I was the only one allowed on that paper according to the hospital. They were all concerned with my mental state and thought that I wouldn't be able to make a rational decision when it came to Mike's health care. Bullshit! I'll make the decisions that Mike would want. There was so much drama between the family, not to mention Suzy and Kathy.

You see Suzy would be up visiting Mike, and a doctor would walk in and think that she was his mother and she never would say that she wasn't. Which really pissed Kathy off. She would come home at night and say, "Well that bitch did it again. She told them she was his mother. *I'm his fucking mother! I've got the forty-two stitches to prove it!*" Forty-two stiches? Who the hell gets forty-two stitches giving birth? I've had two C-sections, and I think combined I didn't have that many stiches.

Anyway, Danielle pulled them both into the bathroom in Mike's room one afternoon, and the conversation went something like this: "I'm telling you two something right now. If *anyone* judges the way my mother is handling this, I'll be on the next flight down, and *no one* will be allowed to see Dad except myself, Elizabeth, Alexandra, and Mom! Do I make myself clear? She doesn't need this right now, so *back off!*"

The two of them were in shock that Danielle was reacting like this. Once again her being daddy's girl. They just stared at her and shook their heads in agreement. My head was in such a fog that the only thing that calmed me was listening to music. One band I came to love is, the Goo Goo Dolls, which my daughter Elizabeth loved as well. There is this one song called "Not Broken" which really fit the situation. I think I listened to that song for a week straight. I drove Elizabeth crazy by constantly listening to it. She would say to me, "You're gonna make me hate that song." I didn't care, it soothed me. Anytime I listened to that song, it relaxed me, and I was able to think more clearly. I think it had something to do with the lyrics in the song. I always felt better after listening to it.

CHAPTER EIGHT

I don't know what day it was; while I was visiting Mike, I noticed what looked to be like a raft that you would float on in the pool on top of him. I was quite confused to say the least. I turned to the nurse on duty and asked her, "What the hell is that and why is it on him?"

She responded by saying, "Oh, it's a heating blanket. His body temp was a little low. So we needed to warm him up a little."

I said to her, "Warm him up? You're talking about a man that sweats when it is sixty-five degrees out. What exactly is his body temp?"

She said that she would take his temperature right then. So after she took his temp, she turned to me and said, "His temp is 96.5. He shouldn't need this on much longer."

So I reached my hand out to feel his head and guess what? He was sweating! I said to the nurse that he was sweating; why does he need this warming blanket still on him? She took his temp again and then said she would turn it off since his body temp was normal. What they neglected to tell me at the time was that Mike was mildly hypothermic. How could they not tell me that? I'm guessing the reason why he was mildly hypothermic was because of the continuous dialysis he was on. Which was drying him out and made his body temp drop.

As I headed back out to the ICU waiting room, I was just shaking my head at what just happened in Mike's room, seeing him with that warming blanket on him. I was still trying to figure it out, but for now I just let it go. I decided to sit down and look through my Facebook account, I noticed that my brother, Brian, in New York had started a GoFundMe account. A GoFundMe account is web page designed to take donations for people that have financial hardships. Examples are funeral costs, hospital expenses, etc. I was in complete shock. As I read what he had written. I began to cry. I was just so touched by what he had written. I noticed that some people had started to donate money. I was just so thankful for this. I showed my daughters this, and they were in shock as well. When I got home, I called him, and I couldn't thank him enough. I really needed the money as I was the only one working with bills to pay. We did have some savings but not enough to cover what Mike's pay did.

I believe it was Friday that I was going to see Mike, and I received a phone call from the surgeon's office. They were telling me that his job needed a return date on the disability claim that I had submitted.

"*What?*" I said. "Are you kidding me? I don't know." She asked me what she should put down. So I said, "I don't know." I was not in the mood for this right now.

She said to me, "I'll just put undetermined for now."

I said to her, "You go ahead and do that."

So the girl said to me that she would e-mail me the forms that needed signing and said to sign them electronically. I thought to myself, *Is this a joke?* I said, "Okay, e-mail me the forms."

So she did. I checked my e-mail, and sure enough the forms were there. I didn't have a clue on how to do it. I asked my daughter, Elizabeth, to help me and she did. All this was done on my cell phone in the hallway of the hospital walking to the elevator. Talk about being overwhelmed? Holy shit! I had been in contact with an HR woman named Antoinette Garcia at Mike's job, and it seemed like they really didn't care about him being in a coma. All they were concerned about was when he was coming back to work. I just couldn't believe it. I mean she knew he was in a coma and so did his managers, Ben Whitman and Roy Dombrowksi. But all they cared about was when he was going back to work.

What I didn't know at the time was that Richard White, who was set to be the new director of engineering at the Star Palace Hotel, where Mike worked, went to visit the hotel and asked where Mike was. He was told that he was out on medical leave. Well you can't believe what he said next. He spoke to the managers in a meeting and said, "Well he should have been terminated by now. If he worked for me in Chicago, he would've been terminated."

He was then informed that they couldn't do that, or they would be facing a lawsuit. This piece of shit turned around and said, "I've done it before, and I'll do it again."

Can you imagine? My husband lay in a coma fighting for his life and this asshole wanted to fire him, and he wasn't even in charge of the department yet. He was just visiting, checking out the new location. What a piece of shit this Richard is. It's a shame that you can't sue someone for being an asshole. My next battle was with Social Security. It's never fun dealing with them as anyone would know who's had to file a claim with them. I hadn't spoken to them yet, but I knew I would be.

We finally got on the elevator and made our way up to Mike's room. I asked the usual questions to the nurses about his condition. They said that he was improving a little more each day. I felt a little relieved, not much. I just sat and stared at him. I was telling him about everyone that came to see him. I told him that everyone in New York was praying for him. I just couldn't imagine my life without him. I just wanted him to open his eyes. After many days of sitting with Mike and praying that he would wake up, I was starting to lose hope. I knew that everyone was pulling for him and that made me feel good. The hospital chaplain came in one afternoon and said a prayer for Mike. A local priest from our church came in too and said a prayer for him. I wasn't ready to be a widow at forty-five. I told everyone that it didn't matter what was wrong with Mike if he was alive. I knew that it was going to be a long, hard road for him. But none of that mattered to me right now. I was up for the challenge.

There was one night where Tom and I were alone in Mike's room, and Tom looked over at Mike and said, "Hey, get up, you're in my spot."

I whipped my head around and said, "Tom, don't talk like that. No one should be in his spot." That comment seemed off colored. It really bothered me that Tom thought he should be in Mike's position. No one should be in Mike's position. Tom and I never saw eye to eye on Mike's care, but that night we did. While we were standing there quietly watching Mike, he started to flail his arms and legs about. We both looked at each other. I was completely freaked out and ran and got the nurse. She came in and said, "Oh yeah, we removed the paralytic today so he's going to do that." That's when we both said, "If he wakes up and realizes that he has a tube in his throat, he is going to try and pull it out on his own. Please restrain him so that he doesn't do that." She assured us that she would.

Danielle headed home early that morning because she had to get back to work. I was an emotional mess to say the least. I really didn't want her to go, but I knew she had to. After all she does have a life in New York, and her job with AT&T was giving her a hard time for coming here. Michelle picked her up and took her to the airport. I hugged her and cried and said that I would keep her posted about Mike's condition. I told her to text me when she landed so I knew she was home safe. After they left, I broke down and cried. Elizabeth reached out and hugged me and said, "Aww, Mommy, everything will be okay. Daddy is going to make it through this." I just shook my head and was barely able to speak. We then got dressed and waited for Kathy and Alexandra to come home from school so we could go up to the hospital.

That night on the way home from the hospital, we stopped at McDonald's for some dinner, and the girls went in to get it. While they were in there, Kathy was on the phone with one of her teacher friends, Debbie Jones, and Kathy was saying, "Oh, I should be home on Monday."

I turned and looked at her and said, "Um, you're with me until Mike gets home. So you better go home and pack more clothes."

She said to Debbie, "Did you hear that? Looks like I'm here indefinitely."

I could hear Debbie laughing on the other end of the phone. The girls soon returned with dinner, and then we made our way home. The smell of the food was intoxicating. I couldn't wait to eat it.

For the last week we were walking around like zombies, barely able to function, much less do anything else. The only time I even left the house was to buy food and go to the hospital. I was due to go back to work on Sunday, and secretly I couldn't wait. I mean I was still filled with guilt about having to go back to work and not being there for Mike, but bills don't pay themselves. I didn't have much of a choice as everything was on my shoulders at this very moment. I wasn't planning on asking for help either. I was going to dip into our savings, which wasn't much to begin with, but it would help.

With the Superbowl coming up on Sunday, I knew it was going to be very hard. Mike was an avid football fan, and even though his team was not in it, he was still looking forward to it. We had even made plans to go to a local restaurant to watch the big game. But that wasn't going to happen now. With Kathy staying with me, the girls and I had gotten back into a somewhat normal routine. When I said normal, I meant not eating fast food for dinner anymore. Nothing about what was going on with Mike was normal, but at least we were going to try and eat healthy.

When I came home from work on Sunday evening, I was surprised to see that Kathy had the game on. She even made some snacks for the girls. She was folding some laundry and cheering along with the crowd. She didn't understand how the game was played, but she did her best. The girls seemed happy, and that was all that mattered to me. Even the dog seemed happier. Even he missed Mike. We all did.

On Monday both Kathy and I were off, and our plans were to clean my apartment and then go up to the hospital to see Mike. Nothing could've prepared me for what was going to happen on that morning.

CHAPTER NINE

Monday morning, we were getting ready to start cleaning and my phone rang. I picked up the phone and said, "Hello."

On the other end of the phone was my daughter, Danielle, excitedly saying, "Daddy's awake! Daddy's awake!"

I was a confused for a moment and said to her, "How do you know this?"

She then told me, "Suzy called me from the hospital, and I was able to talk to him for a few minutes using FaceTime!"

Why didn't Suzy call me, why did she call Danielle? Go figure…I'm his wife. Needless to say, I was elated that he was awake.

Still holding the phone, I ran into the living room screaming, "He's awake! He's awake!"

Both Kathy and Elizabeth looked at me like I was crazy. Kathy, with a perplexed look on her face, asked me, "How does Danielle know Mike is awake if she's in NY?"

I told her that Suzy was there with Mike when he woke up and called Danielle and told her. This did not sit well with her at all. Her reaction went something like this "That bitch! She's not his fucking mother I am! What the fuck is she doing up there with him!"

You see Suzy was up there every day to see Mike. She would rub lotion on his feet and wash his face. She did whatever she could to keep the peace since Danielle spoke to her and Kathy. This made Kathy very angry. I told her, "Maybe you should've taken some time off from school, and then you could've been up there everyday too! So instead of standing there and complaining go get dressed so we can go and calm down ok?" I didn't even take a shower. I could've cared less about what I looked like.

The previous Saturday afternoon, Suzy asked me why I wasn't wearing makeup. I said to her, "Do you really think that I give a shit about what I look like right now? He's in a coma and has no I idea what I look like. So, please, just leave me alone about wearing makeup, okay?" She really didn't say much after that. I was starting to think that she wanted me to meet someone else. It really annoyed me.

All I knew was I had to get up there to see Mike. I got dressed as fast as I could, we all did so we could go. We arrived at the hospital and took the elevator up to his room. When we got there and we finally saw him, he looked so confused. Suzy was there, and she was getting ready to leave. I hugged her and thanked her for being there for Mike. She became very emotional as she was leaving. He was so groggy and had no idea what was going on. I was just so happy to see him with his eyes open. I asked him if he knew who I was. He kind of nodded his head. He couldn't speak due to the tube still being in his throat. We were all elated that he was awake, but we knew he still had a very long road ahead of him.

He was just lying there, looking around like he didn't know where he was. I just kept telling him that I loved him and that he was going to be okay. I was going to do whatever it took to make sure that Mike didn't have to go back to work to soon. I was even willing to work two jobs if necessary. I asked the nurse when they were going to take the tube out of his throat. She said that all depended on Mike and how well his breathing was. So I crossed my fingers and prayed that his breathing would get better. I felt like I was in a dream because I thought I would never see him alive again.

My youngest daughter was still in school and had no idea that Mike was awake. Kathy had said that she would go get Alex from school and bring her up so that she could see Mike awake. I was grateful that she would do that. I was so overwhelmed that I couldn't think straight. I sent out a group text to our friends and family, letting them know that Mike was awake but still had a long road ahead of him. It had only been twelve days that he was in a coma, but it felt like month. I was mentally, emotionally, and physically drained from everything. But I was glad that he was awake.

CHAPTER TEN

Tuesday morning before Kathy went to work, she went up to the hospital to see Mike. That's when she called me and told me, "He clocked me!"

I couldn't help but laugh. I said "What?" You see Mike had these mittens on his hands that resembled Mickey Mouse's hands.

She said, "He wanted water, but because the tube was still in his throat, he couldn't have any. So he clocked me!"

Laughing, I asked her, "Are you okay?"

She said, "Yeah, but I can't believe he did that."

As I hung up with her, I couldn't stop laughing. When I told Tom what happened later that day, he replied, "Well about time one of us did."

I just couldn't wait to hear his voice. I would only have to wait one more day. By Tuesday afternoon his breathing improved to the point where the tube was able to be removed. But Mike being Mike, he was trying to pull it out himself. I kept telling him to stop, but he was so uncomfortable with the tube being in his throat. The doctor came in to check to see how well his breathing was. He told me that he was breathing well but had me look at his belly. I asked him why.

He said to me, "Do you see the way his belly is moving and shaking? Well it must look steady, like he's not struggling to breathe. Right now, it looks like he is."

I tried to explain to the doctor that he was agitated and that if they just removed the tube he would calm down. But they wouldn't listen to me. I pleaded with them to remove it, but they wouldn't budge. What could I do? I sat down in the chair next to Mike and just started crying. I was just hoping that they would remove it in the next few days. Mike was very upset, and I tried to reassure him that the tube would be coming out soon.

Wednesday morning Elizabeth and I were walking down the hall to his room and the respiratory therapist stopped me and said to me, "He was extubated this morning."

I looked at her excitedly and said, "He was!" I just started running with Elizabeth to his room. The next thing I heard was Mike saying, "I can speak! I can speak!" I ran to his room, and Suzy was there of course, and Mike looked at me and said, "I can speak." The first thing I did was take his hand in mine, and I asked him if he knew who I was. He looked at me a little confused but then after a few seconds he said, "Baeba." You see that's a nickname he had been calling me for years. As you can imagine I was ecstatic that he remembered that. I looked over, and on the bed tray by the window was a Darth Vader bust that Tom had gotten for Mike. I went over and picked it up and showed it to Mike and asked him who it was.

He took it out of my hand and held it for a few seconds. I was a little apprehensive that he wouldn't know who it was. He just held it for a few minutes and stared at it. He asked me who got it for him. I told him that Tom did. He twirled it in his hand and then said, "Darth Vader?"

I said "Yes! Yes! You remembered!" We sat there and watched TV with him for a while. He was so thirsty, but I couldn't give him any water. I paged the nurse, and she said he could have ice chips. Just having the tube removed, his body was not ready to handle any regular food yet. He had to start slow. The nurse brought the ice chips and said to spoon-feed it to him like he was an infant. He was getting frustrated, but I told him that it wouldn't be long before he was able to eat regular food. He had an oxygen mask on to help him breathe easier. I knew that it would be weeks before he could eat normal again. I continued with the ice chips.

I don't know what time it was, but I know Alex was up there, and the infectious disease doctor came in and was checking on Mike. He was asking him some routine questions like his name, date of birth, etc. He then looked at Alex and asked him if he knew who she was. Mike says, "Of course, I do. It's my oldest daughter, Danielle."

That's when Alex said to Mike, "No, Daddy, I'm Alexandra not Danielle."

The doctor gave me a concerned look but then smiled and said to me, "It's okay. He just came out of a twelve-day coma. Let's give him some time for his memory to come back." I was a little apprehensive but again I put my faith in that the doctor knew what he was talking about. We left sometime around five thirty and went home to have dinner.

That same day Suzy came up to visit, and she was chatting with Mike. I guess they must've taken blood from Mike because he kept asking Suzy if his tests were back. She understood him to say, "Are my testicles black?" So she said, "Well I don't know lift sheet, so I can see them."

Mike said, "No, no, are my tests back?"

Suzy started hysterical laughing because she now realized what he was asking her. She said to him, "No, no, they're not back yet."

CHAPTER ELEVEN

On Tuesday night his father and brother came up to see Mike. While they were sitting and talking with Mike, out of nowhere, Mike asked them, "Was I shot?"

Tom looked at him and said, "No, you weren't shot. You just had surgery." His father said the same thing to him.

Mike said to both, "You're lying to me!"

They both said, "No, we're not!"

Mike said again to them, "Stop fucking lying to me! I know was shot!"

They were both laughing because Mike kept insisting that he was shot. They reassured him that he wasn't shot and that he had surgery and was in a coma for twelve days due to major complications from it. You see the reason, Mike thought he was shot was because while in his coma he had a vivid dream that he was at Disney with our youngest daughter Alexandra. He dreamt there was a shooting there, and he jumped in front of her to protect her and that's how he was shot. I guess his subconscious was playing tricks on him. He was still unable to distinguish reality from his dreams. When they came up dinner was being served. His father thought that he was being helpful and decided to feed Mike. Well he started pumping the food in him.

Tom said, "Dad, you can't feed him that fast. He can't handle that much food at once."

His father said, "Nonsense. He needs his nutrition. He hasn't eaten in twelve days."

All the while Mike was waving his arms at his father, trying to tell him that he was gonna be sick. He was making the motion with his hands that he was going to throw up. Tom said, "Dad, he's trying to tell you he's had enough food."

His father said, "No, he's not, he's saying he wants more." Next thing you knew, Mike projectile vomits all over his father. He was like, "Uggh, OMG. He puked on me!"

Tom sat back with his arms folded and said, "See, I told you." While laughing his ass off, Tom said, "Dad, you were in the Navy, you should be able to handle this."

His father said, "Yeah, but I never had to deal with puke" He got up and ran into the bathroom to wash his hands. Mike kind of just shrugged his shoulders while Tom kept laughing.

Tom said, "I told him to stop, you think he would've listened." It was all over his sheets. It was a mess. Tom had to page the nurse so that they could come in and clean Mike up. After the nurse got Mike all cleaned up, they left for the night. They were both tired after working all day.

On Wednesday we went up in the afternoon to see Mike. Since it was Ash Wednesday, I said a little prayer that Mike would continue to get better. The nurse said that he had eaten a little that day. I was extremely happy about that. While Elizabeth and I sat there with Mike, the hospital chaplain came around and asked if we were Roman Catholic. Seeing as it was Ash Wednesday, he asked us if we wanted ashes. Mike looked at me then looked at the priest and said, "Sure. A little can't hurt."

After the priest left, we continued to watch TV. We were talking and out of nowhere Mike said, "Do we have a case?"

Elizabeth and I just looked at each other with confused looks on our faces. I replied, "A case? Against who?"

Again he said, "A case against the idiot who tried to kill me."

I said, "Who tried to kill you?"

He replied, "The dog."

I said to him, "The dog tried to kill you?"

At this point he's becoming agitated and said, "Yes, the dog who tried to kill me!" Well as you can imagine, Elizabeth and I were hysterically laughing.

So Elizabeth said, "You mean Chase?. Who by the way is our family dog?"

He again said, "Yes! The idiot who tried to kill me!"

So Elizabeth turned around and said, "Well you may have tried to kill him. But he didn't try to kill you." We both got a kick out that and laughed.

I guess his bowels were functioning normal again because a little while later he turned around and said to me, "I've shit the bed!"

I couldn't help but laugh and looked at him and said, "You did what?"

He again said, "I've shit the bed."

I said, "Okay. I'll get the nurse."

The nurse came in, and he said to her, "Hi! I've shit the bed."

The nurse said, "Indeed you have. I'll get you cleaned up."

So with that Elizabeth and I went down to the cafeteria and got some dinner…the only thing worth eating was Subway. So we got sandwiches. After we finished eating dinner, we went back up to Mike's room, and he was all cleaned up. He was having his first physical therapy session, and he looked over at me as I walked in and said, "Look what I can do."

I said, "Wow, that's great!" The therapist had him lifting just the top half of his body to build his arm strength. Seeing as he couldn't walk yet, I was just happy to see him at least lifting the upper half of his body. We stayed a while longer and then we went home for the night. With everything that was going on, it was nice to see Mike getting his sense of humor back. If you knew him, you would understand.

The next morning at around 8:00 a.m., Kathy called me to tell me that Mike was out of ICU and had been moved to another room. I was elated! She had said to me that he had fallen. I was a little alarmed at first. You see none of the nurses had told him that he was in a coma for twelve days and was unable to walk unassisted. He had fallen because he was getting up for a walk to go find his father. He had no concept of time. He couldn't tell or read time. We came to find out later that he in fact really did hurt himself. But more on that later. He was becoming agitated. He had come so far, and if he had really hurt himself, I would've been devastated.

She told me he was okay and that the nurse hollered at him and told him that he couldn't get out of bed just yet. Kathy proceeded to tell me that when she got up there that morning, Mike was telling her this wild story of how all night this older gentleman, who was down the hall from him, kept saying, "Help me. Help me" He had finally had enough and screamed, "Yeah, I'm gonna help you. I'm gonna hit you with a baseball bat! *Shut the fuck up!*"

The nurse came in after he said that and thanked him for saying that because they couldn't. Kathy looked at him and said, "Michael, why would you say that?"

He said, "I didn't sleep all night because of his fucking screaming!" Then he told her that there was a woman who was giving birth, and when she finally had the baby, they held the baby up and kept smacking the baby on the ass. I'm not sure what language they were speaking, but from what Mike said, he thought it was Arabic. Every time they hit the baby, he or she would cry. Again Mike was annoyed with this and he screamed, "*You hit that baby one more time, I'm gonna come in there and smack you!*" Quietly they closed the door. I told her that I would be up there when Alex was out of school.

It was later in the afternoon after Alex was out of school, that we headed up to the hospital to see Mike. A good friend of ours, Robert Volpe, called me on my cell phone to tell me that he was up there and waiting to see Mike. He had been up there when Mike was still in his coma, and now he wanted to see Mike awake. Unbeknownst to me, Mike had been taken down to have the dialysis port removed from his groin, and they were going to put it in his chest. The reason they were relocating the dialysis port was because his groin was becoming infected. Robert called me on my cell phone and asked me what room Mike was in. I had told him, and he was like "He's not in there." I thought, *Okay, I don't know where he is then.*

I arrived at the hospital and was on the elevator up to Mike's room when my cell phone rang for the one hundredth time. I answered it, and it was Kathy on the other end. "Where the hell are you?"

I said. "I'm on the elevator up to Mike's room, why?"

She said, "Okay, well hurry up. They need to do a minor procedure on Mike."

I asked her "How minor?" That's when she told me that they were relocating the dialysis port.

She then said, "I'll have the nurse meet you there."

They thought Kathy was Mike's wife. She told them she wasn't his wife, that she was his mother. They kept saying that they were in a time crunch and needed to do this procedure. Mike was adamant that he was not letting them touch him until I got there.

Kathy told them, "Tell everyone to call home and let them know you're all going to be home late."

As I got off the elevator, I almost walked into Rob. He handed me an envelope and said, "I don't like GoFundMe. Take this." I hugged him and thanked him. Inside the envelope was one-hundred-dollar cash. I was stunned. He said, "Listen, I've just finished a twenty-four-hour shift and I am exhausted and need some sleep."

Rob is a cop in Tampa and was helping in Orlando. I again hugged him and apologized for Mike not being there. He said not to worry about it and that we would talk soon. I told him that I would keep in touch. No sooner than I said goodbye to Rob, a nurse came around the corner and said, "I'm looking for the wife of the patient in room 222."

I said, "That's me."

She said, "Follow me."

I told the girls to wait in Mike's room while I followed the nurse. As we made our way down to where Mike was, I asked her if he was okay.

She said, "He's very nervous, but he's okay."

I said, "Well I can't blame him considering what he's been through the past two weeks." She nodded her head in agreement. When we got off the elevator, I saw Kathy standing there, waiting for me. She immediately came over to me, took me by the hand to where Mike was lying on a gurney.

Mike turned his head and like a child looked up at me and said, "I'm scared." He then lifted the sheet to show me his privates and said that it looked like a paint by numbers down there. He was shaking something awful. My heart was breaking. He didn't want any more surgery. I couldn't blame him. He then started to cry which really tugged at my heart.

I reached down to him and said, "Look at me. Do you trust me?"

He looked up at me and nodded his head.

I said, "Okay, if you trust me then everything will be okay."

At this point we were both crying and hugging, and I told him that I loved him and that I would see him soon. I kissed him on the head and then turned to follow Kathy back up to his room and wait for him to come back up.

CHAPTER TWELVE

When we got back to his room, the girls asked how Mike was and what was going on with him. They were anxious to see him. Pretty soon his father arrived along with his brother. I don't know how long we were sitting there, but the doctor who performed the procedure on Mike stuck his head in and said that it was done and that Mike was doing well and would be up soon.

I breathed a sigh of relief. I thought to myself, *Will this nightmare ever be over?* While we sat there waiting for Mike to come back, I was talking with his dad and I mentioned to him that Al and Gina had sent Mike flowers.

He said, "Really?" I pointed to them sitting on the nightstand.

I guess Tom wasn't too happy about this because he turned around and said, "Nobody sent me anything when I was in the hospital for my kidney transplant."

I said. "Yeah, well were you in a coma for twelve days fighting for your life? No, you weren't. So don't you dare stand there and compare yourself to Mike right now. I understand what you went through was serious, but now is not the time to be doing this." Not another word was said. Everyone fell silent after that. With all the drama between Kathy and Suzy, this was the last fucking thing I needed right now.

At around 5:00 p.m., Mike finally came back up from the OR. He was awake and chatting away with the doctor. As he was being rolled in, I heard him say, "I'm back."

As soon as I saw him, I breathed a huge sigh of relief. He was looking around at his surroundings, and he looked a bit confused. I asked him, "Are you okay?"

He said, "This isn't my room."

I looked at him and said, "Yes, it is."

Again he said, "No, it's not."

"Yes, it is," I said again.

He then asked, "Where are my flowers?" He was referring to the flowers his cousins, Al and Gina, had sent him. They were in a pink vase with a pink ribbon around it that said "Get Well."

I pointed to them and said, "They're right there on your night table."

He turned around and looked at them and said, "Okay." He seemed content after that. He talked about the procedure that had been done and how he woke up in the middle of it and said, "I'm awake." And the surgeon told him, "You're going back to sleep."

They soon brought some dinner for him, and he was famished. I fed him slowly. He still wasn't used to eating at this point, so I had to spoon-feed him little bits at a time. Of course, he was not happy about this. But once again I assured him that soon he would be eating normally again. His father and brother left at some time around seven. Kathy was tired and wanted to leave and Elizabeth did too. Alex became increasingly upset and didn't want to leave. So I told Kathy to just go home with Elizabeth and that I would be home soon. She asked me if I was sure and I said yes. So Alex and I stayed a bit longer.

We just sat there watching TV with Mike. Alex lay next to him in his bed. While watching TV Mike casually turned around and said, "I've shit the bed again." He became all embarrassed about it.

I said to him, "It's fine. It's not a big deal. I'll just call the nurse to come clean you up." I went out to the nurses' station and told them what happened. When the nurse came in to clean Mike up, Alex and I went down to the cafeteria to eat something. We decided on Subway. As we chose what sandwich we would eat, we said that we would get banana peppers on the sandwich in honor of Mike. Mike loved banana peppers on sandwiches. I know it sounds silly, but it made us feel better. When we got back to Mike's room, we saw that he was all cleaned up. We sat a little while longer, and then we headed home for the night. Thank God tomorrow was Friday.

CHAPTER THIRTEEN

Friday at noon Elizabeth and I headed up to the hospital. When we got there, we noticed that they were serving lunch. He was very thirsty, and all he wanted was water. I opened the bottle of water on his tray and was giving him little sips. He wanted to drink it from the straw, but the doctor had told me just to spoon-feed it to him. he was not happy. He pleaded with me. "Please, can I drink it from the straw?"

What could I do? So I let him do it. I told him, "Drink it slowly." Well he started sucking down the water like it was the last supper. I pulled the straw out of his mouth and said, "You're going too fast."

He asked for more and I said no. Suddenly he started coughing. I asked him, "Are you okay?"

The next thing I know he threw up all the water he just drank. After he wiped his mouth, he looked at me and said, "I guess maybe I should've used the spoon?"

I said to him, "You think? Yes, use the spoon."

I had reached out to some former coworkers that Mike had worked with to let them know what had happened to him. It was around three thirty and Oscar Hernandez, who was Mike's former chief at Sunshine Resorts, called to check on Mike. I told him that Mike was out of the coma but still had a long road ahead of him. He asked me to please stay in touch and that when Mike was feeling up to it, he wanted to see him. I thanked him for calling and said that I would let Mike know that he called.

It was around four thirty when one of Mike's coworkers came up to visit him. It was Miguel, who we've known for some ten years. When this all happened, they all wanted to come see him, but I told them that now wasn't a good time and that I would let them know when it was a good time. Miguel brought Mike some puzzle books and some Star Wars things. He hugged me and said that I was a good wife. They chatted for a while even though Miguel knew that he was still out of it due to the coma. Kathy was there and chatting with Miguel as well.

Mike's friend, Michael, called and spoke on the phone with him. Of course, Mike was telling him this wild story of how he was the captain of the Nautilus and trying to save Captain Nemo. We were also the Clauses trying to save his mom. Which brings me to the morning when all he as saying was "It's my fault she's dead. It's my fault she's dead." When Kathy got there that morning, the nurse almost didn't let her in.

She asked Kathy, "Who are you?"

Kathy said, "I'm his mother!"

The nurse said, "You're alive?"

Kathy said, "Yes I am! Why do you ask?"

The nurse said, "He's been saying all morning it's his fault you're dead."

Kathy said, "Well I'm not!"

It was quite comical to say the least. I believed all the drugs were playing with Mike's mind. But if you ask him to this day, he believes it was all real and that it happened.

I was finally starting to see the light at the end of this long, dark tunnel when in walk these two doctors and asked if I was Mike's wife. I said yes, I am. They proceeded to tell me that he was going to be transferred to Hill View Rehab Center.

I said, "*What!* Today?"

She said, "Yes. Didn't someone speak to you?"

I was becoming agitated and got a little loud with her "*No!* No one did! He just came out of a coma two days ago! How can they move him already?"

She responded by saying, "Well you'll have to call his doctor to find out more information."

They told me that at around 5:00 p.m. an ambulance would be coming for him. I felt like I just got punched in the stomach. I just stared at them and asked them what Hill View Rehab Center was.

They explained that due to his pneumonia they could take better care of him there. Were they throwing him out of the hospital? This was too much. So I picked up the phone is his room and called Dr. Lopez and told him to please come to Mike's room.

About ten minutes later he was there. I asked him what Hill View Rehab was. He said that it was a rehabilitation center. I asked him, "Is Mike well enough to be transferred?" He assured me that he was and that he would get better care there than if he stayed here. I felt a little relieved.

Miguel stayed a little while longer with his girlfriend. They left around five that afternoon. Mike's father headed up to the hospital when he was finished with work. He decided that Mike needed a shave and asked me if it was okay if he did so. I said sure. Who am I to argue? He even brought up a shaving kit.

His father turned to me and said, "What do you think Anne, should I give him side-burns?"

I laughed and said, "Sure why not. He'll never know."

I was thinking about Mike's reaction when he would finally be able to see himself again in a mirror. It would be very funny. After he finished shaving him, dinner was being served. So his dad started to feed him aggressively. Kathy told him to go slow. But did he listen? No.

Once again he was like, "He needs to eat."

Kathy said, "Yes, he does but slowly, don't shovel it in like that."

His father wanted to leave after he was done feeding him. Mike didn't want him to go. He was hanging on to him like a little boy would do. He kept saying, "Don't go."

But his father said, "I have to go. I must help Suzy with her medication. I'll be back tomorrow to see you." Finally Mike let go of his hand and his father left.

We sat there and watched TV and waited for the ambulance to come for him. We were getting restless and hungry. I finally went out to the nurses' station and asked, "When is the ambulance goanna get here?"

She said that she would find out. She came back and said that it was on its way. So again we continued to wait. We sat there for hours, waiting and waiting. I again went out to the nurses' station; this time I wasn't so nice. I screamed at her and asked again when it was coming. I got back to Mike's room and sat down at the foot of his bed.

All of a sudden I heard Mike say, "I'm going to be sick."

Now I don't do puke. So Kathy grabbed the basin on Mike's tray and held it under his mouth. Next thing you knew he's puking everything that his father fed him. I felt so bad for him. I had to turn around while Kathy cleaned him up. By now I was highly annoyed that the ambulance wasn't there yet. It was dark now, and I was exhausted and had work the next day. I again went out to the nurses' station and inquired about the ambulance.

She replied in the most unconcerned way, "It's coming. They have other stops you know."

Well I was not going to put up with that. Not after dealing with what I was dealing with this last week. I crossed my arms, looked at her dead in the face, and said, "Why don't you get off your ass and call someone and find out what the hell is taking so damn long!"

Kathy came out into the hall where the nurses' station is and said, "*She better not be charged for this ambulance taking so long!*"

I think the nurse was terrified at this point and got up and went to call to see what was taking so long. We both headed back into Mike's room. He was trying to get up out of bed. I said to him, "What the hell are you doing?"

He looked at me and said, "I have to pee!"

I said to him, "That's what the catheter is for!"

He was becoming argumentative at this point. He kept asking why he couldn't get out of bed. I explained to him that he was in a coma for twelve days and his legs were very weak. But he kept trying to get up. I told him that the catheter would damage his privates if he kept on trying to get out of bed. He kept trying.

Finally I said to him, "If you ever want to have sex with me again, you'll stay in this bed and not get up!" I knew it sounds harsh, but I was at my wits end! He was like a five-year-old. He just wouldn't stop!

He just looked at me and said, "Okay."

I felt his head and he felt feverish. I thought, *Oh great, now he's running a fever.* I took his temperature and sure enough he had a low fever of 99.9. He thought that he was going home but I knew he wasn't. All day he kept saying to everyone that he was going home. He told me that I was to go buy pastina and Sprite. Oh, and he needed Epsom salt to help his privates to feel better because the nurse told him that it would help. I knew that because he was running a fever, he may not be transported to the rehab center. So I tried to keep him calm and get him to stay in bed. I knew he was frustrated. Shit, I would be too! After all he hadn't been able to walk in two weeks! That's all he wanted to do was get up and walk around.

Finally after what felt like an eternity of waiting, the ambulance guys showed up. They knew by looking at him that he wasn't well enough to travel just yet. They were getting his vitals, and sure enough he was still running a low fever. They explained to me that they had to wait until his fever went down then he would be able to be transported. Which I completely understood. I was mentally, physically, and emotionally drained from being up there all day. I knew Alexandra was home alone, and once again I was torn; do I go or do I stay? So I headed out to the nurses' station and told the nurse that I was leaving and to please call me as soon as Mike was being transferred. I went back to Mike and kissed him and told him that I loved him and that I would talk to him in the morning.

I got home and showered and settled down for the night. The nurse called me at ten to let me know that Mike was being transferred to the rehab center. While Mike was still at the hospital, they were continuing to give him a hard time about being taken to the rehab facility. You see Dr. Anjali was refusing to release Mike due to his low fever, which really made Mike more agitated than he was. If he wasn't released soon, his fever would have skyrocketed.

Finally Mike said to the nurse, "Call my father if he doesn't want to release me."

Five minutes later she came in and said, "Okay, he's good to go."

The guys took him to the ambulance, and as they were loading him in, Mike said, "Can you put the sirens on?"

The guys were so nice to him, they said, "Sure, buddy, whatever you want." He was like a little kid riding in the ambulance.

When he arrived at the rehab center, they started taking pictures of him to make sure that he had no bruises or bedsores and to make sure that he hadn't suffered any abuse from the hospital. As they were doing this, he peed himself. He was so embarrassed, but the nurse said not to worry about it and that she would clean him up. After they cleaned him up, he fell asleep for a while.

He has this wild dream that he was a train conductor and lost control of the train and crashed into the wall. Well now he was awake. Once again Mike had soiled himself and was being cleaned up. They washed him for the first time in about a week. They gave him clean pj's and wrapped him a warm blanket to keep him warm. The nurse had given him a sedative to relax him. So what did he do? He spent the night trying to get out of bed and get a dragon hallmark ornament that was hanging on the wall. Much to his dismay he never did get that ornament.

CHAPTER FOURTEEN

On Saturday morning I called the rehab center to check on Mike. They transferred me to the ICU, and I spoke with the nurse on duty. She said that he was doing okay and that he had a bit of a rough night, but it was to be expected.

I asked, "How rough?"

She said, "Well because he had the catheter in for so long, he peed himself, but I told him it was okay and not to worry."

I asked her if I could bring up regular clothes for him so that he could be a little more comfortable. She said that would be fine and just no undershirts due to his IV in his neck. She also told me that he was going to be in a regular room very soon and that him being in the ICU was a precaution due to his pneumonia.

My next phone call was to his dad. I told him that Mike was doing okay and he had a rough night but otherwise was in good spirits. He asked the name of the facility he was in and I told him. I told him that I would be unable to go up as I had to work. Of course, I was being judged for going to work and not going to see Mike. But I didn't really give a rat's ass on what anyone thought. I had two children to take care of and bills to pay. I told his father to please stop by my house and pick up some clothes for Mike. I had packed some underwear, pajama pants, and some socks.

Kathy said that she was going up as well and would let me know how Mike was when she got there. I took a shower and got ready for work. His father came and picked up the bag I packed and went to the rehab center.

Sunday was Valentine's Day, and I was just so happy Mike was alive and getting better. He kept hounding Kathy to get me flowers and candy for Valentine's Day. I told him that there was no need for any of that. My gift was that he came back to me.

Kathy said to me, "Oh my god, if I don't get you flowers, I'm never going to hear the end of it!"

So on Sunday night when I got home from work, there on the table was a small vase with flowers in it and a small balloon. I was stunned to say the least. I quickly took a picture of it and put it on Facebook for everyone to see. I had brought a big heart-shaped balloon to Mike for Valentine's Day. His dad brought him balloons too. Kathy took us out to dinner on Valentine's Day. We really enjoyed ourselves. It was the first time in two weeks that I was relaxed.

On Monday Mike called me and asked, "Hey is anyone gonna come see Bob today?"

I thought, *Who in the world is Bob?* What I didn't know was Mike had been watching the *Minions*, and one of them was named Bob. I guess he really liked that character. I never knew he liked the *Minions*, but there was a lot that changed with Mike; I just didn't know it yet.

I was getting back to a somewhat normal routine. I was starting to feel like that this nightmare was coming to an end. Mike was in a rehab center continuing to get better, and I was very happy. The rehab center was very nice. They allowed us to bring up food for Mike. He had his own private room, which was nice. There was a gentleman who was down the hall from him, and he called him fried chicken guy because that's all he ever ate. All Mike wanted was pastina and Sprite. Kathy would prepare it at my house and bring it up to him on the weekends because she worked during the week. Tom would bring him food and so did his father. Mike wasn't a fan of hospital food, but who was? So it was nice that we were able to bring food to him. At least I knew that he would eat, and I didn't have to worry. All he enjoyed from the rehab center was the cold tea and pizza. Now Mike couldn't walk on his own yet, but he was trying.

One morning he had to go the bathroom, and he had buzzed the nurse several times. But there was no response. After he couldn't wait any longer, he took matters into his own hands. He strategically placed the pads that they had underneath him in bed on the floor, and very slowly he made his way to bathroom. He carefully pulled himself up on to the toilet and was finally able to go. He also made a mess in the process. There was pee everywhere. He had no control of his privates just yet due to the catheter being in for so long. He did the best he could to clean himself up. Now came the tricky part—getting back to his bed. His legs were still very weak and unable to support his weight—not that he was heavy. So he pulled the string over the toilet and waited.

This time the nurse came charging in and saw him on the toilet. She said to him, "How did you get in there?"

He said, "I used the pads! I called you several times, but you didn't come, so what was I supposed to do? I'm tired of pissing and shitting in the bed!"

She was very mad and went and got the nursing supervisor. They both came back, and she told the nursing supervisor, "I'm not cleaning that mess up!"

The nursing supervisor asked Mike, "How did this happen? How did you get in here?"

Again Mike explained how he got to the toilet. He said, "I called her several times, but she never came! What was I supposed to do?"

The nursing supervisor told the nurse to help Mike get cleaned up and clean up the mess and next time to respond quicker. That was the last time that happened. They put the alarm on Mike's bed so they would know if he got out of bed.

CHAPTER FIFTEEN

Later that day Tom came up to see Mike. He had sliced up some apples for Mike to eat. As Tom was slicing up the apples, he proceeded to tell Mike what happened when he went to buy Trix cereal for him. Now you see the rehab center isn't in the best of neighborhoods. Well Tom went into what you would call a bodega; it looked a little sketchy, but he figured, *What the hell they may have Trix cereal.* Anyway he went in and asked the clerk at the counter, "Do you have Trix?"

All of sudden he heard a woman's voice say, "I've got a trick for you, darling. Why don't you come over here and I'll show you?"

Tom looked at her and said, "Not that kind of trick, the cereal Trix."

She responded by saying, "Darling, my tricks are better."

He said, "No, thank you." He just turned around and left.

Mike was hysterically laughing and couldn't believe what Tom was telling him. They ate some apples and just relaxed and watched TV. Mike had dozed off for a while, and when he woke up, he said, "Oh, man, I peed myself again."

So Tom said, "What do you mean peed yourself again? Just call for the nurse to come help you."

Mike said, "No, dude, you don't understand. This isn't the first time. She's mean, she won't answer."

Tom said, "*What?* Go ahead, call her."

So Mike called for the nurse, and she came. As she was helping him get cleaned up, she looked at Tom and said, "He is so needy. He's always calling for me."

Well Tom lost it. He looked at her and said, "He wouldn't be here if he wasn't needy! Everyone in here is needy! At least give me the urinal so I can help him if you don't want to!"

The nurse just stood there in shock and just handed Tom the urinal and turned and left. What they didn't realize was that Mike popped a stitch and was leaking fluid, not peeing himself. This was discovered when they came in to bathe Mike that night. After she left Mike turned and said to Tom, "That right there is why I call her Nurse Ratched." He was referring to the mean nurse in *One Flew Over the Cuckoo's Nest*. They both laughed. Tom was getting tired and had some errands to run and told Mike that he would back tomorrow.

The next morning a nurse came by Mike's room to see if he wanted to go outside for some fresh air. Mike said, "Sure, that would be great." He was looking forward to getting out of his bed for a while.

The nurse brought a wheelchair in and helped Mike get into it. She wheeled him outside into beautiful sunshine. As he was sitting there, he said to the nurse, "You're lucky I don't have sneakers on otherwise I would make a run for it."

She chuckled and said, "Not on my watch."

Later that day when I went to the rehab center to see Mike, we were walking to his room, and we noticed that he wasn't there. I immediately panicked. I started to walk around in the hallway, and that's when I noticed a nurse walking with him with the wheelchair right behind him in case he couldn't walk anymore. I was shocked and happy at the same time.

He looked up at me and said, "Hey, babe, look I'm walking!"

I said, "I know! That's great, keep it up!" He was really trying hard but getting frustrated at the same time. I told him that it's okay Rome wasn't built in a day. He kind of relaxed and sat down in the wheelchair and wanted to go back to his room. We all went back to his room and sat down and relaxed. Lunch was being served, and Mike was very hungry. But he wasn't eating much. I asked him what was wrong. He said that he still felt like he had the tube in his throat. I told him that he had to try to eat something otherwise he wouldn't be able to come home for his birthday. "This food is awful. I can't keep eating this shit. Can you bring me food from home?"

I told him that Kathy would bring him up pastina for him. "Is there anything else that you would want?"

He said, "Get more Trix cereal, Goldfish crackers, and more apples."

Guess I had some shopping to do. But it was okay. I would've done anything to make sure he was eating. Mike's dad had brought up Gold Peak iced tea so that Mike would have something to drink other than the water at the rehab center.

On Saturday, while Mike was waiting for Kathy to bring up his food, he kept saying, "I'm hungry. I'm hungry." He called her and asked her when she was coming up, and she told him very soon. So instead of eating his breakfast that was given to him, he decided to wait for Kathy. Tom had arrived a while later to visit with Mike.

Mike asked him, "Where's Mom? She's supposed to be bringing me up my pastina?"

Tom replied, "I don't know. I thought she was already up here. Look, here are some eggs. Why don't you eat them?"

Mike said, "I don't like eggs."

Tom said, "Since when? Everybody likes eggs. Look, there's some meat here. Why don't you eat it?"

Mike said, "What kind of meat is it?"

Tom said, "Looks like a sausage patty."

Mike said, "Well, why don't you try it?"

Tom said, "I don't like sausage patties."

Mike said, "Well, I don't like eggs."

Tom looked at Mike and said, "It seems we've reached an impasse for you having breakfast. Why did you order eggs if you don't like them?"

Mike said, "I didn't. That's what they gave me."

Tom said, "Well, at least eat the potatoes and toast."

Mike said, "Fine. But I still want my pastina."

While Mike was eating his potatoes and toast, he called me and asked me where Kathy was. I said, "I don't know. I thought she was up there already. I'll call her and find out where she is."

She had told me that she had to go home and get something, and then she was going to bring Mike up his food. When I reached her on the phone, she told me, "I had to go home and wait for a package for Tom."

I was furious with her. I said, "WHAT! Why couldn't Tom have waited for it? The rehab is on my way to work. Had I known you were going to be waiting for a package, I would've brought Mike up his food. But now it's too late!"

She said to me, "I know. Tom should do a lot of stuff on his own. I'm only going to wait ten more minutes, and then I'll bring Mike his food."

I called Mike back and told him.

He said, "A package? What package? Hey, Tom, why is Mom at home waiting for a package for you? Why couldn't you wait for it?"

He said, "What? I didn't ask her to wait for any package. I don't know what she's talking about."

Mike had these patches on him to monitor his heartbeat. One morning after a nice bath, clean sheets, and clean pj's, he was very relaxed. He was sitting in a chair in his room just watching CNN, and he was bored to death. Suddenly the nurse came running in and asked Mike if he was okay

He looked up at her and said, "Yeah, why?"

I guess the nurse was talking to the person who was monitoring him and said, "Yeah, I'm in Papsodero's room. He's fine."

Whoever she was talking to said, "Well his heartbeat is very low."

The nurse said to Mike, "Your heartbeat is very low."

Mike said to her, "Well that's because I'm very relaxed and I'm watching CNN and I'm very bored."

The nurse told him to do something to raise his heartbeat.

Mike said, "What do you want me to do?" The nurse shrugged her shoulders. So Mike started flapping his arms like a bird and said to the nurse, "There, is that better?"

The nurse started laughing and asked whoever was monitoring him if his heartbeat was high enough. I guessed it worked because the next thing he knew the nurse that was monitoring him said, "Yep, that'll due."

Everyone got a good laugh out of that.

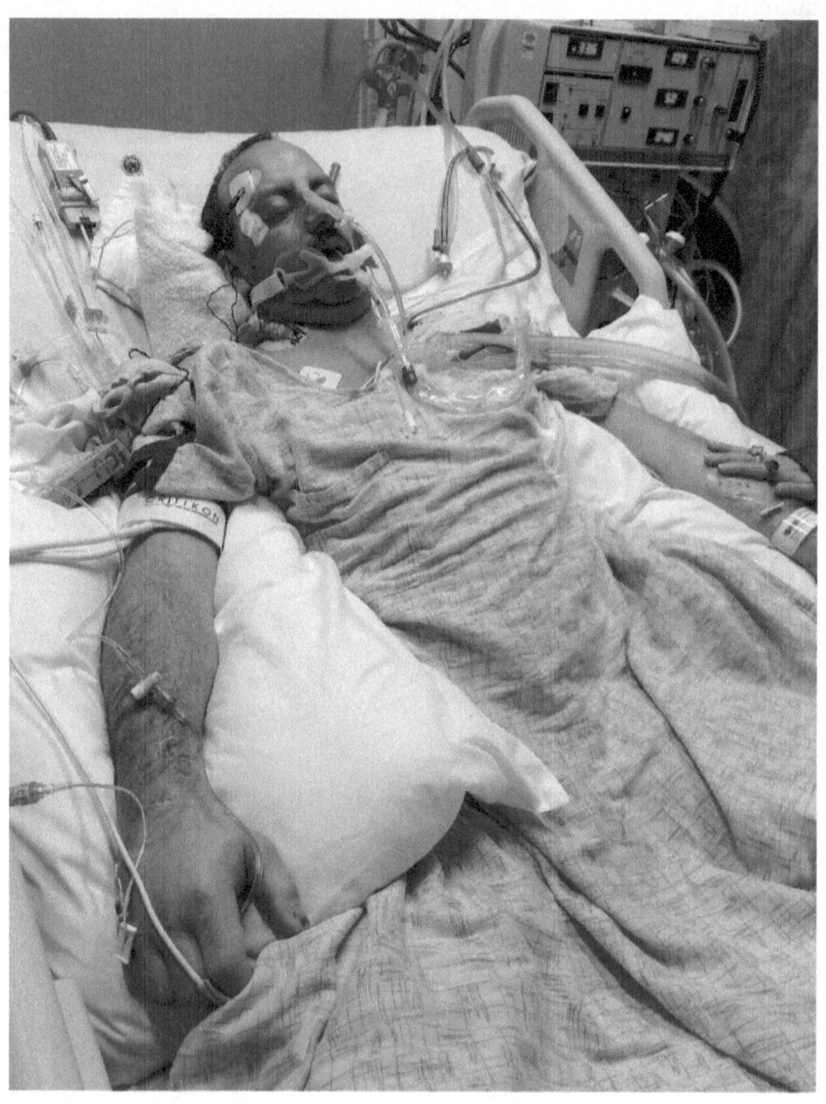

Mikes first day in the coma. It would be 2 long
weeks I would see him like this.

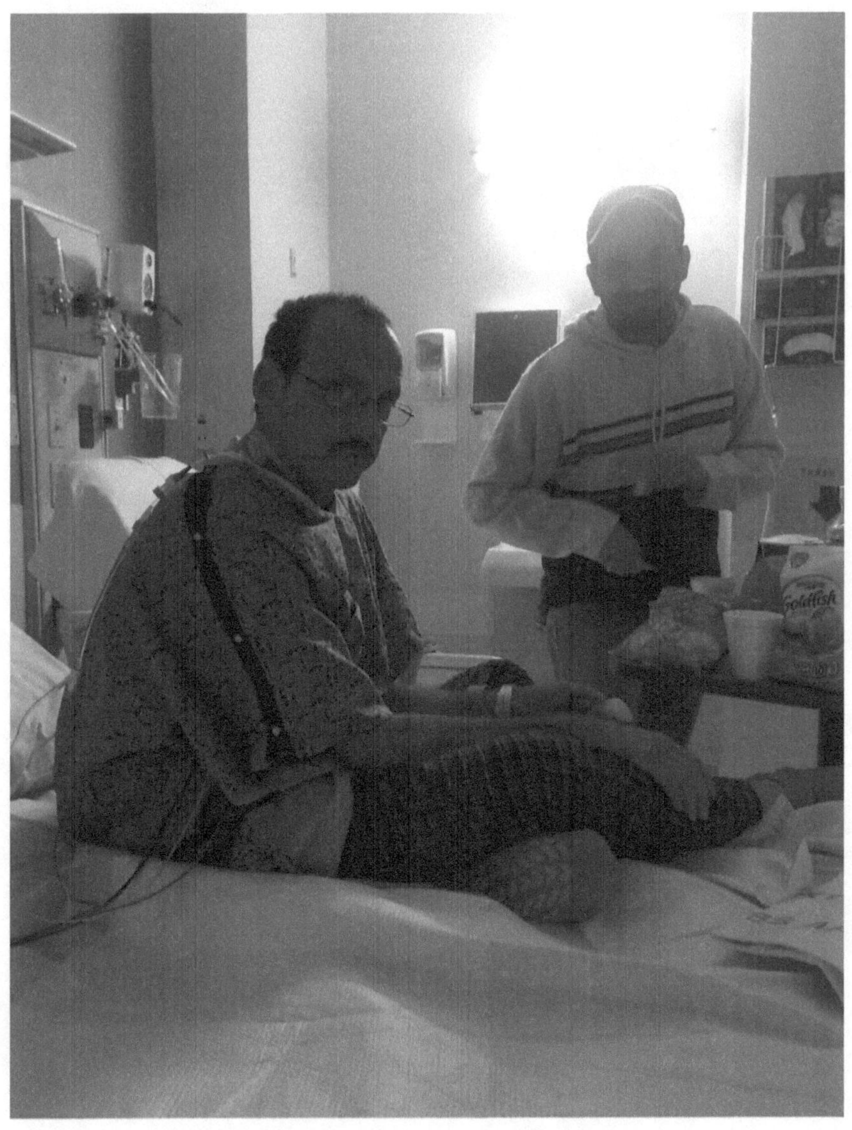

Mike and Tom enjoying some apples. Tom
brought apples for Mike all the time.

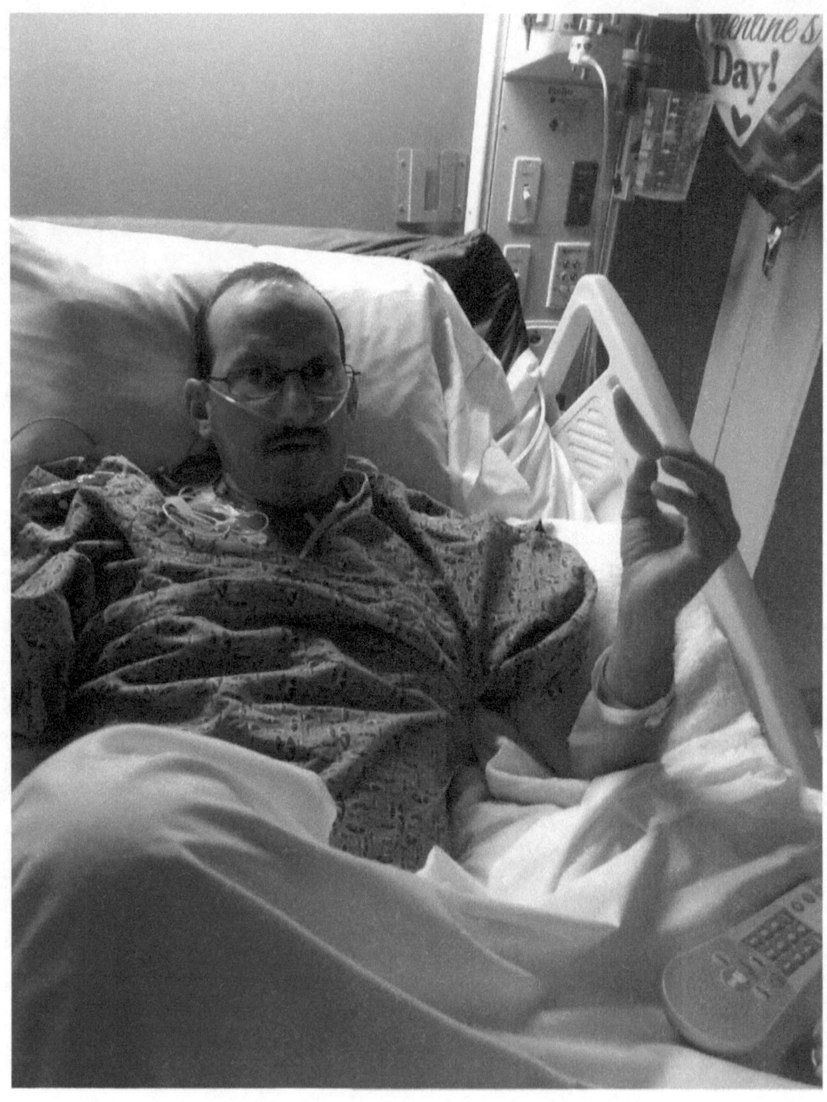

Best Valentines Day present ever. To see him like this
was amazing. I never thought I would again.

CHAPTER SIXTEEN

Mike was starting to get around a little better each day. So one day while I was at the rehab visiting him, he made his way to the bathroom. He hadn't seen himself in the mirror in a while. So as he was standing in the bathroom looking at himself in the mirror, he was a little surprised at what he was seeing. He yelled out to me, "Hey, who the fuck shaved my mustache? And how the fuck did I get sideburns?" I started to laugh like crazy. He yelled again, "It's not funny. Why is my mustache so thin?"

I said, "Dad shaved you a few times. He wanted to give you sideburns." Now Mike loves his mustache and doesn't let anyone touch it.

"Why did you let him shave me?"

I said, "The hair on your face was so long it was disgusting! I don't know how to shave a face, so I thought who better to do it than Dad."

He said, "But why did he have to go so thin on my mustache?"

I said, "He wanted to clean it up."

While sitting there with Mike, he asked me, "Hey, who was playing music for me while I was in the hospital?"

I looked at him in amazement. I said to him, "You were in a coma, how did you hear music? Tom played AC/DC for you. Was that who you heard?"

He said, "No." He was insisting that he heard the Queen's song "Show Must Go On" and "Every Breath You Take" by the Police.

I asked him, "Are you sure that's what you heard?"

He said, "Yes, I'm sure."

I was shocked to say the least. I mean I've heard that coma patients can hear you while in a coma, but I never knew they could hear music. It makes sense though.

Mike had started physical therapy and was doing well. He was also being taught how to read, write and tell time again. These simple everyday things that we take for granted. Mike had to relearn again. Things seemed to be progressing well. I was hoping that he would be able to come home soon. His birthday was coming up, and I knew he wanted to be home by then. Every day I would visit with him, he would ask me, "When can I go home?" It broke my heart, but I just didn't have an answer to that. I kept telling him soon. I finally received a paycheck of Mike's and of course these idiots sent him a paper check instead of directly depositing it. Now seeing as he couldn't even write, I had to hold his hand so he could sign the check, so I was able to deposit it. These idiots kept asking when he was returning to work. I felt like telling them *never*! But I couldn't do that. They were becoming extremely annoying, and if I told them that it would've been the end of his job right then.

On February 17 he had to go for another MRI to see how his intestines were doing. He was given the contrast so that when they did the MRI, they would be able to see clearly. Well he got sick from the contrast. He called everyone's phone number that he could remember. But no one answered. He finally reached Suzy. She then sent me a direct message on Facebook to call Mike right away. He just wanted someone to come and help him get out of the rehab center. I was confused as to why he didn't call the house. So I called the rehab center and spoke to him.

When I finally spoke to him, I asked him why he didn't call the house. He said, "I did call the house, but no one answered." This only frustrated him more. He also told me that all he wanted to do was go home. I told him, "We must wait for the results from the MRI and then we'll talk to the doctor about you coming home." He relaxed a little and said okay. He was still feeling nauseous after the MRI. Maria, the nurse, came back and told him that she had the results of the MRI. He was a little backed up or, as she put it, "full of poo." She finally gave him a shot for the nausea. She assured him that it would help him feel better. Well not only did he not feel like puking anymore, he now had to "go." And go he did. The nurse, Maria, noticed that his progress had stopped moving forward and instead was going backward. She made it her top priority to make sure his progress would move forward again. She told him that there would be no physical therapy or walking today. The number of drugs that he was being given just made him sleepy.

February 22 is Mike's birthday as well as his father's birthday, and I went up to see him in the morning because I had a doctor's appointment that afternoon. That afternoon his father brought up a red velvet cake for him. Mike looked at the cake and said to his father, "What the hell is this?"

His father said, "Well it's red velvet cake."

Mike said to him, "But I don't like red velvet cake."

His father looks at him and said, "Well Elizabeth likes it."

Mike said, "Yeah, but it's not her birthday, it's mine." His father told him to eat it anyway. Mike said, "But I don't want to eat it. I don't like red velvet cake." He was acting like a child; it was quite comical to say the least. They sang "Happy Birthday" to Mike and reluctantly he had a piece of red velvet cake. After they had cake, his father asked, "Hey, have you heard any news as to when you will be going home?"

Mike said, "Actually, I have I should be going home on the twenty-fourth."

His father replied, "Are you sure you're ready to go home? You're still very weak. Maybe you should stay a little longer?"

Annoyed Mike said, "Dad, I'm tired of hospitals, I'm tired of the food, and I just want to be home in my own bed. If they say I am ready, then what's the problem?"

His father said, "Okay, I won't say another word about it."

We finally received the news that Mike was going to be coming home on February 24. I was so happy. He was still very weak, but he was well enough to come home. I was so excited that he would finally be coming home. I was given instructions by the nurse that Mike was going to continue at home his physical therapy. They were also going to send a walker to the house so he could use it to get around.

Mike was like a child on Christmas Eve. He was giving me a list of things he wanted to do the day he came home. I said to him, "Hey, hold on a minute, you're still very weak. There's no way you'll be able to walk around that long." He was very insistent that he would be. I explained to him that he was going to need a lot of rest.

The night before he came home, I was dusting our bedroom and I was singing the song "I'm Coming Home," but instead of "I'm coming home" I substituted it to "He's coming home." I was just so excited that he was coming home. I wanted everything perfect for him. I was planning on picking him up at twelve thirty and then running a few errands and then taking him straight home. The air seemed lighter, the mood was uplifting, and everyone was just elated that he was finally coming home. Mike called me and told me to be there at 9:00 a.m. sharp. I said to him, "There's no way they are going to release you that early, but I'll be there."

The day had finally arrived! Elizabeth and I arrived at the rehab center at 9:00 a.m. sharp because Mike thought he was being released first thing. We had to wait until the doctor discharged him and for him to get all his medications before coming home. Mike was becoming anxious and just wanted to go home. I assured him that we would be leaving soon. They also had to remove the dialysis port before he was able to go home, as well as have the IV removed from his neck. I knew that this wasn't going to be easy for him as he didn't like needles, let alone someone removing one from his neck and his chest.

The nurse came in and asked him, "Are you ready for me to remove your IVs and your dialysis port?"

He looked over at me with this terrified look on his face. I said to him, "Just relax, everything is going to be okay. Once this is done, the doctor will come in with your discharge papers and we will be able to go home." The nurse then removed everything and said that she would go get the doctor.

Finally the doctor came in and gave me all the instructions for his at home care. I helped him get his sneakers on and helped him sit in a wheelchair. After thirty days in the hospital, he was finally going home. The nurse advised me to go get my car and bring it to the entrance. So I did just that so Mike wouldn't have to walk that far. I pulled up and went around to the passenger side door and opened it. The nurse helped him get in the car. Elizabeth was sitting in the back seat and was just so happy to see Mike.

As we left the parking lot, Mike said to me, "We have to go to CVS and get a shower chair for me and then we have to go to Publix and get pastina and Sprite and then home."

I laughed and said, "How much do you think you can do? You were just in the hospital for thirty days, don't push yourself."

He looked side-eyed at me and said, "I can do anything."

I said, "Oh yeah? We'll see about that."

CHAPTER SEVENTEEN

When we got to CVS, I parked the car and went to help Mike get out of the car. As he stepped out of the car, he was a little shaky.

I asked him, "Are you sure you can do this?"

He assured me that he could. We made our way into CVS, with Elizabeth on one side and me on the other to hold Mike up. He was walking slow. I told him that I would go get him a scooter, but he was too proud for that. So we walked very slowly, and we made our way to the entrance.

He looked at me and said, "Maybe you should've taken me home?"

"I wanted to, but you insisted you wanted to come. When we go to Publix, I'm getting you a scooter. I don't care what you say." He sheepishly agreed.

We made our way to the back of CVS to the pharmacy area. I took Mike to the seating area and had him sit down while I asked where the shower chairs were. The girl pointed me in the right direction, and I found them. I purchased one and then we left. We then went to the supermarket to get Mike his pastina and Sprite as well as drop off his prescriptions. I had gotten a scooter for him, and of course at first he was resistant, but then he was okay with it. He was driving that thing like it was a hot rod. He looked at me and said, "I feel like an old person." I told him not to worry about it, that he had just gotten out of the hospital after thirty days, and it was fine. We paid and then went home.

All he wanted was a nice, hot shower and a nap. As we walked through the door, our beagle, Chase, was so happy to see Mike. I let him out of his crate, and he came charging right over to Mike. He was so weak that he couldn't even bend over to pet him. I helped

Mike into the bedroom and had him sit on the bed while I got the groceries and shower chair out of the car. Once everything was in the house, I put the shower chair together. I set it down in the tub, and I helped Mike get undressed. I helped him into the bathroom and into the tub. As he walked by the mirror, he caught his reflection in the mirror. He just stood there in shock. I guess I didn't realize how thin he was.

"I want to weigh myself."

"No, don't, you'll be upset."

"Stop telling me what to do and help me stand on the scale"

So reluctantly I did. He stepped on the scale and nearly fainted. He weighed an astonishingly 136 lbs.! He was 5 ft. 9.5, and before the surgery he was 167 lbs. He had lost 31 lbs.! He was not happy about this at all. Surprisingly he just said to me, "I guess I'll gain it back eventually."

While he was in the shower, Chase all but climbed in the shower with him. He laid on the floor beside the tub, waiting for Mike to get done. He wouldn't leave his side. After he was done, I helped him get dressed. I made him his pastina for lunch. I got him settled on the couch so he could rest. I had to go back to Publix later to pick up all his medication. Alex was at school but knew that Mike was coming home and couldn't wait to see him. Mike asked if we could get pizza for dinner.

I asked him, "Are you sure you can handle that?"

He said, "Absolutely."

"Okay, we'll see."

Kathy was still staying with us and would probably be going home over the weekend. She was anxious to see Mike too. She was at work and would be home around four thirty that afternoon. I called her and told her that Mike was home. I also told her that I would be ordering pizza for dinner. She was like, "What? Can he handle that?"

"He says he can, so we'll see."

Alex came home at around 4:05 p.m. and ran right to Mike. "Daddy! How do you feel? Are you happy to be home?"

"Yes, I'm very happy to be home. I get to sleep in my own bed tonight."

I ordered the pizza and it came at six. We ate, and Mike was really enjoying it. I asked him how his throat felt. He said that it was okay. After we ate, I had to go back to Publix and get all Mike's medications. Kathy said that she would take care of the laundry for me. I took Alex with me.

While in Publix we ran into a neighbor of ours, Carla, as we were leaving. She had heard about what happened to Mike from her daughter who went to school with Alex. She asked me how everything was going and how Mike was. I told her that he was finally home, but he still had a long road ahead of him. "I'll be taking a leave of absence from work to stay home and take care of him. I'm just glad he's alive."

She said that if I needed anything, to let her know. I thanked her, and we said our goodbyes and headed home. When we got home, I noticed that Kathy was gone. I asked Mike where she had gone.

He said, "She aggravated me, so I told her to leave."

"*What!* After all she did for us? Why would you do that?"

"She was telling me what to do, and I didn't like that, so I told her to leave."

"Well what was she telling you to do?"

He said, "She was telling me what to eat and what I should or shouldn't do. I disagreed and told her that I'll do what I want, and she got mad and left."

"You are unbelievable. She was probably looking out for you." Yup, he was back to normal.

CHAPTER EIGHTEEN

Later that night I called my job's HR hotline, to let them know that I would be taking a leave of absence. They said that it wouldn't be a problem and they would let my manager, Chris, know. I couldn't believe that it was that easy. I was so relieved. I could now focus on taking care of Mike. I sent a group message to our friends in New York and let them know that he was home. All our family knew he was home. Everyone was very happy for us. A few of his friends wanted to call and talk to him. He did speak to some of them. He was still weak and would get tired very easily. We were in bed by 9:00 p.m.

Let me start by saying that it was very hard to sleep that first night he was home. Even though he was so weak, he still wanted to be intimate with me. I had to blow him off. He was having horrible nightmares and woke up screaming a few times. He kept yelling for the nurse. I had to keep telling him that he was home so he would relax. Eventually I was able to get some sleep, not a lot but some.

In the morning we got up and I made Mike some breakfast. He was barely able to eat. He had little to no energy. He ate what he could and went right back to bed. He took his pills, which were a lot, and just relaxed in bed. He watched TV and listened to music. I did some laundry and cleaned the house a little. We really couldn't go anywhere. Eventually Mike got out of bed and sat on the couch. Sometime that afternoon Mike's former chief engineer, Oscar Hernandez, from Sunshine Resorts called. You can't believe the story he told us.

The phone rang, and Mike answered it. "Hello?"

Oscar said, "Dude, you don't know how good it is to hear your voice. Oh my god."

Mike said, "What the hell are you talking about?"

Oscar proceeded to tell him that a few weeks ago, he was in Miami visiting his mom and gets a phone call from this guy David who worked with both Oscar and Mike. The phone call went something like this.

"Hi, Oscar, this David. How's everything with your mom? Listen I just got a voice mail message from Mike's wife. Jesus, I don't even know how to tell you this but Papsodero passed away on Friday."

Oscar said to him, "*What?* What do you mean he passed away? OMG, he was so young. How did this happen?"

David said, "I don't know, she didn't say. All the message said was that he passed away Friday."

Oscar said, "Holy shit. Okay, I'm leaving tomorrow."

On Saturday the Admin Lillian, from Sunshine Resorts, formed an e-mail and sent it to the entire engineering department saying, "We regret to inform you that Mike Papsodero, former HVAC Engineering Manager, has passed away. We are taking donations for a floral arrangement to give to his wife. Thank you in advance."

Now everyone who used to work for Mike read this and was devastated. No one wanted to call me because they felt that I needed time to make the arrangements. Oscar told everyone, "I'll call Anne on Monday and find out all the details." At this point everyone was crying and in shock and still trying to wrap their heads around this. Oscar purchased the biggest floral arrangement he could find and has everyone sign a condolence card for me.

That Sunday morning, they found out that it was a different Mike that passed away, not my husband. It was a Mike who worked at a different Sunshine Resorts location. Everyone was relieved that it wasn't my husband. Not that it wasn't sad about the other Mike, it's just that they didn't know the other Mike. They all knew my husband very well. A lot of the guys even worked for him. Now Lillian doesn't work on weekends, so they had to wait until Monday to retract the e-mail she had sent out.

When she found out, she said, "OMG, how did this mix up happen?"

Can you imagine they all thought he was dead? And the reason for the confusion? The wife of the other Mike never left her last name when she called David. She just said that she was calling to let David know that Mike passed away on Friday. So for the whole weekend they thought that Mike was dead.

After hearing this, Mike said to Oscar, "OMG, are you serious?"

Oscar laughed and said yeah. He said, "When you're feeling up to it, come for a visit and I'll show you the e-mail. I'm just glad that you're okay." They spoke a few more minutes and then hung up.

CHAPTER NINETEEN

For the next few days we just stayed in the house so Mike could rest. We really couldn't do much. Mike had to call the Social Security office so that they could start processing his claim. He also had to call his short-term disability people to finish that claim. Neither of us were working, and we needed for one of the two claims to be approved. The only thing that I had was the GoFundMe account which had $4,950 in it. I was in the process of getting that withdrawn and deposited into my checking account. At least that would help us until Mike's short-term disability claim was approved. I was thankful that my food stamps were approved. At least I had money to buy food. It was tough.

Mike was going to be starting his at home physical therapy on Monday. He was really looking forward to it. He was still having a hard time getting around and was becoming frustrated with himself. I explained to him that the therapy would help him become stronger. His walker had come, and I would take him outside and have him walk around the block with it. He complained about having to use it, but he did. It was quite nice. It had a seat, so if he got tired, he could sit. It had hand brakes to make stopping easier, and it had a basket underneath it for carrying groceries. I was hoping that the therapist would use it for his therapy. I didn't know what the therapist was going to do. I guess we would find out on Monday.

On Monday morning at 11:00 a.m., the therapist came to our house. He sat down in the living room with Mike and asked him several questions about his health history. He informed us that as well as being a physical therapist, he specialized in psychotherapy, which meant that Mike would be able to talk to him about certain things that he felt he couldn't talk to me about. He started to have Mike do some exercises to build up his leg strength as well as his upper body. He did them reluctantly, but he did them. The therapist was scheduled to come once a week for about one to two hours a day or however long Mike was able to tolerate it. Mike seemed to be enjoying the exercises he was doing. We even purchased some dumb bells so that Mike could do some arm exercises on his own.

It was one week later, a Wednesday night, that Mike started to experience abdominal pain again but on the opposite side. We had just finished eating dinner. We had pasta that night, and I thought pasta never bothers Mike. He told me that he was going to lay down and rest to see if the pain would subside. I thought to myself, *Oh no, not again.* He was in excruciating pain. I assumed that he was constipated, so I gave him a laxative. I even called the surgeon, Dr. Lopez, and he agreed with me for giving him the laxative. He managed to get some sleep, not a lot.

So on Friday morning we were back in the ER again, but not County General. This time we went to Kissimmee General. After what happened in January, I vowed never to go back there. When Alexandra left for school that morning, she looked me dead in the eye and said, "Dad better be home when I get home from school!"

I couldn't blame her. After everything that we went through for the last thirty days. I replied, "I'll do my best to make sure he's home."

We left shortly after to go to the hospital. When we arrived at the hospital, Mike became extremely upset and just didn't want to be there. I told him that we really didn't have a choice. We needed to see what causing his abdominal pain. I called his mother to let her know what was going on. She told me that she was on her way. They took him immediately. We sat in the triage area for a while. Eventually the doctor on call came to examine Mike. She asked Mike some routine questions about his health. I explained to her about the last thirty days. That's when she said he would need an MRI, and then we would know what was causing his pain. I sat there holding Mike's hand and told him that everything was going to be okay.

Inside, though, I wasn't sure. I was starting to have flashbacks of the last thirty days. I tried my best to put on a happy face, but I was finding it hard to do so. Kathy arrived shortly after. The nurse brought Mike the contrast that he was supposed to drink, which by the way was disgusting. The contrast made Mike violently ill. Thank God for Kathy because I don't do puke. Boy, did he get sick. I've never heard him get that sick. After about thirty minutes, they came and took him for his MRI. I told the nurse that Mike was just violently ill and that there might not be any contrast left in his system. She said that it was okay and it shouldn't be a problem. So off he went for his MRI.

I waited with Kathy for him to come back. He came back about twenty minutes later. We waited for the doctor to come back with the results. She finally came back. She told us that Mike had what seemed to be a bowel blockage. She asked Mike who his surgeon was at County General and then said we should go back there. I asked her why we needed to go back there. And that's when she dropped a bomb on us. She proceeded to tell us that Mike was going to need surgery again and that it would be best if the original surgeon performs it.

"Absolutely not! Do you understand that he will die this time? He is much too weak to undergo another surgery!"

She said, "Well I'm just telling you what I see on the MRI."

I responded by saying, "And I'm just telling you he's not having another surgery. Is there another surgeon here?"

She told me that the attending surgeon would be in to talk with me. After she left Mike looked at me and started crying and said that he was scared and didn't want any more surgery. I couldn't blame him. The surgeon came in and told us that it did look like Mike in fact had a bowel blockage but he was not rushing to have surgery just yet. He was going to let Mike rest overnight and see how he was feeling in the morning. I let out this huge sigh of relief. I don't think that I could've handled another surgery.

Both Kathy and I left around 8:00 p.m. Kathy said that she was going home, but I couldn't handle this by myself. I called my cousin, Caroline, and was bawling into the phone and asking if she could come down. She was unable to but told me that she would call Kathy and make her stay with me. Caroline called Kathy and told her, "You better stay with her! Tom is a grown man and can take care of himself! So don't give me that bullshit that you have to be there for him."

And guess what? She stayed with me until Sunday afternoon. I was relieved that I wouldn't have to go through it alone.

CHAPTER TWENTY

The next morning Mike called me, and he sounded much better. I asked him how he was feeling. He said that he was feeling much better, and to get rid of all his medications. I asked him why, and he said that they were making him sick. I told him that I couldn't do that. That's when he told me what happened the night before. First the laxatives that I had given him finally worked. He proceeded to tell me that at 11:00 p.m. the night before, he had to go and called the nurse that was on duty. The nurse brought him one of those kidney-shaped plastic basins. Mike took one look at it said, "What, are you kidding me? You're gonna need three of those! Just unhook my IVs and let me use the bathroom."

So the nurse did that and helped him to the bathroom. And boy did he go. He went three times that night! I asked him, "Do you have a room yet?"

He said, "No. I'm still waiting in the triage area. I'm hoping to have one soon."

I asked him, "Have you slept at all? Have you eaten anything?"

He told me that they were going to start him on clear fluids after another MRI and that he barely slept. I told him that I would be up soon. I was hoping that by the time I got there, he would be in a room. I was grateful that he was feeling better, but we still weren't sure what was causing his abdominal pain. I really didn't want Mike to endure anymore surgery. His body was much too weak.

When I arrived, Kathy was already there. Both of us just couldn't believe that Mike was back in the hospital. We both were chatting with Mike. He seemed in good spirits, considering what took place over the last thirty days. I had called his father and told him that Mike was back in the hospital. He was in shock and asked what happened. I told him that we were still trying to figure it out. He said that he would be up to see Mike after he was done with work.

The nurse was in and out, monitoring Mike's blood pressure. So far so good. I knew once his father came up that would change. His father had told him not to be in a rush to go home from the rehab center, but Mike was just so done with being in the hospital. I was just hoping that this would be a quick stay. He was becoming antsy and wanted to go home. I told him that once we knew what was causing his abdominal pain, we would be able to go home. I also told him that if he didn't calm down, his pressure would go up and then he would be in real trouble. He quickly stopped. We talked about planning a vacation in the summer. Everyone in New York wanted to see him.

It was around four when I left. I wanted to be home for Alex and reassure her that Mike was okay. I was anxious to get the mail as I was waiting to hear a response from Social Security. I was hoping that things would go my way. I still wasn't back to work yet, so we really needed this to go our way. The only thing that we had was Mike's short-term disability payments, which weren't much. I still had some of the GoFundMe money left so that was helping pay the bills for now. But that wouldn't last forever. As I pulled into the parking lot, I was praying for a miracle.

My heart was pounding in my chest as I was getting the mail. The first thing that I noticed was a card from my mom. When I opened it, there was a check for one hundred dollars in it. She wrote a lovely note, saying that she was praying for Mike, and even though it wasn't much, she hoped that it would help me out. I was so thankful for this. I thought to myself, *Well, at least there is some good news.* And there it was. An envelope from Social Security. I quickly tore it open. Beads of sweat were forming on my forehead as I started to read it. Denied! I was pissed. I was screaming and crying because I just couldn't believe that he got denied. I just kept saying how are we going to survive this! As soon as I got in my apartment, I picked up the phone and called Mike in the hospital, which I knew I shouldn't have done but I did it anyway. And as soon as he picked up the phone, I started screaming at him about how he got denied.

He said to me, "Babe, where am I? I'm in the hospital. What do you want me to do? It's Friday afternoon at four. If I'm home on Monday, we'll call together, okay?"

I calmed down and apologized to him. "I'm sorry for screaming at you. I'm just frustrated with all this. No one is helping me. I'm the only one working, and I was really hoping that this came through. Yeah, I appreciate that Mom was staying with us, but she didn't offer to help with any of the bills."

He said to me, "I understand, and I love you for how strong you have been throughout this whole thing, and we will get through this like everything else that has been thrown at us, okay?"

"Okay," I said.

The nurse came in to check his pressure, and as you can imagine it was high. She told him to hang up with me and relax. So he did just that. She was not happy that his pressure was so high. It was 180/80. Mike's father got there around five thirty, and all he did was tell Mike how he should eat farina or oatmeal and that it was good for his heart and that Suzy made the best farina around.

Mike said, "I don't like farina or oatmeal, so I'm not eating either of them."

But his father kept insisting that he try it. At this point the pressure cuff started up again, and his pressure hit 190/85. The nurse took one look at that and went back into Mike's room and turned to everyone in the room and informed them that if they don't stop aggravating her patient, she's kicking everyone out.

At this point Mom said, "I'm not leaving."

The nurse said to everyone, "My patient has been through enough and he is not having a stroke on my watch! I will have everyone trespassed!"

The nurse told her that she'll have her trespassed. Dad then said he's leaving and for Mike to relax, that everything will be fine, and he'll see him when he gets home. Kathy stayed with Mike until he got a room late Friday night.

CHAPTER TWENTY-ONE

Saturday morning Mike called me and told me that he finally got a room. *Thank God*, I thought. The thought of him spending one more night in the ER was pissing me off to no end. I asked him if the doctor had been in to see him yet. He said that he was still waiting for him to come. He was sent for another CT scan, this time without contrast. I was really hoping that he didn't have to have another surgery. I told him that I would be up soon to see him because I had some things to do around the house. He asked me if I would stay the night. He told me that the room was nice and big and that he felt like he was in a hotel. I said that I would have to think about it. I know that it sounds mean, but I was over hospitals at this point.

I got there around two, and I have to say that I was really impressed with this hospital room. It was nice and big, and he was the only person in the room. It didn't look like your ordinary stale hospital room. He even had Netflix on his TV! The doctor came in a short time later and spoke with us. He told us that he looked at the first CT scan that Mike had, and he didn't have a blockage. He informed us that some of Mike's scar tissue had come loose and wrapped itself around his intestine and that was the pain he was feeling. He also told us that when Mike had pooped, that did the trick and the scar tissue unwrapped itself. He told us that Mike would be able to go home today. He was just waiting on the second CT scan to confirm what he found on the first one. Once he had the results, Mike would be able to go home. Mike was so excited and couldn't wait.

As soon as the doctor left, Mike asked me to help him to the bathroom. He wanted to shower and get dressed. I said to him, "Whoa there, mister, we don't even have the results yet. It could take a while. So just calm down. Okay?" He started to sulk like a little kid. I said, "No one said you couldn't take a shower, but we don't know how long it'll be before we get the results of your CT scan."

I helped him in the shower. He was still very weak and was very unsteady on his feet. After he showered, he wanted to go for a walk down the hall. He was starting to feel his oats now. I helped him get dressed, and we went walking. He was happy that he might be able to go home today. As we walked up and down the halls, he was very chatty, and his mood completely changed. He was talking to all the nurses and even some of the patients! He was telling me all the things he wanted to do once he got home. He became tired and wanted to go back to his room. As I helped him get back in bed, there was a knock on his door. I was hoping that it was the doctor with the results of CT scan. To my dismay it wasn't. It was a nurse with a menu, asking what Mike would like for dinner. I was like, "Wow, he gets to choose from a menu. I'm impressed."

I was getting hungry myself. After I helped him pick out something for dinner, I went down to the cafeteria to get something to eat. I was really getting sick of hospital food. But at least there wasn't any Subway because I was sick of Subway. As I looked at the menu, I saw burgers and thought, *Ooh, I could really go for a burger right now.* Just thinking about it made my mouth water. I placed my order and waited for my food. I guess I must've been gone a while because Mike called my cell phone and said, "Where are you?"

I said to him, "I was waiting for my food and I saw Mom, and she ordered some food for herself and the girls. I'll be up soon, okay?"

He said to me "Yeah, she came with the girls just after you left."

I said, "Okay then, just relax and I'll be up soon. Is there anything you might want? How about I bring you a cookie? They have these jumbo chocolate chip cookies. I'll bring you one."

"Okay," he said.

We finally got our food and headed back up to Mike's room. When I walked into Mike's room, he had Netflix on, and by this point I knew that he wasn't going to be able to go home tonight, which soured his mood. So I went out to the nurses' station and asked if there was an update on the reading of Mike's CT scan. She said that she would contact the doctor. We started eating our food while we waited for the doctor to come. The doctor finally came in at eight and said that they hadn't read his CT scan yet and that it might be early morning before they could. I told the doctor that he had the CT scan early in the morning on Saturday and I wanted to know why the hell it was taking so long. He said that when he asked why, they told him that by the time they got to it that was the time for them to go home. Well this didn't sit well with Mike at all. I thought he was going to explode.

Kathy and the girls decided that they were going to leave. I said that I was going to leave at around nine. The doctor said that maybe the results would be in tonight, but he couldn't guarantee it. Mike wanted me to spend the night with him, but I didn't have any clothes with me. In the back of my mind, I knew his motive for wanting me to spend the night with him. He wanted to have sex with me. He had a private room and I guess he figured, "Hey, I'm already in the hospital so if anything were to happen, I could just page the nurse." Like I said before, Mike is anytime, anywhere kind of guy, so his thinking was what the hell why not. Not that I would have done it, but you never know. I told him that I would be up first thing in the morning. I knew he was disappointed and frustrated, but my only thought was his wellbeing and to have him home again.

CHAPTER TWENTY-TWO

Sunday morning Mike called me at around eight thirty and asked when I was coming up. I told him that I was having breakfast and that I would be up. I finished my breakfast, showered, and then I headed up to the hospital. I was really hoping that they had the results from the CT scan so Mike would be able to go home. When I got up to Mike's room, he was already dressed.

I asked him, "Why are you dressed already?"

He replied, "The results came in very early this morning, and everything is normal. The nurse said I was a little backed up, and I told her that's because the CT scan was taken over twelve hours ago, and I had gone since then."

"Well what did she say to you after you told her that?" I asked.

He replied, "She said that I would probably be going home later this morning. We just have to wait for the doctor to sign off on the paperwork."

I was very relieved after hearing that. I asked him if he was up to going to BJ's to shop when we left. "Of course, I am," he said. I laughed when he said that. I was picturing him driving around on the scooter all through BJ's.

The doctor came in to speak with us and told us that Mike would be going home soon. Mike was delighted to hear that. The nurse came in a short time later with all the paperwork for me to sign as well as a little care package for us to take home. The care package contained a container of soup, some apple juice, and crackers. *Very impressive*, I thought. The soup was enough to feed all four of us.

As you can imagine from reading about Mike, I made him go home first and have some of that delicious soup he got from the hospital for lunch, and we then went out to BJ's to shop. Of course, when we got to BJ's he wouldn't listen and get a scooter; typical guy response: "I don't need that, I'm fine." Until about a half an hour of walking around gathering up groceries, he became very fatigued. I then insisted that he get a scooter. The girls and Kathy were with us, and after some browbeating, he finally relented and got a scooter for the rest of our shopping trip. Once he was on that scooter, he took off like a bat out of hell! My youngest daughter, Alex, was riding with him. I had to chase after the two of them. It was like a three-ring circus in BJ's. All you heard was me saying, "Hey! Get back here!" The two of them thought it was the funniest thing making me run around BJ's and chase after them. I was working up quite a sweat.

Upon returning home we all insisted that Mike should rest as we unloaded all the groceries. But would he listen? *No!* He thought he's superman until he crashes. He just had to help, and then reality gave him a swift kick in the ass. The disc that was herniated gave him a sharp shooting pain down the back of his left leg, and that's when he finally said, "Okay, I think I'll stop now."

I said to him, "See, I told you this was going to happen. But would you listen No! Now go sit on the couch and relax or do you want to go back to the hospital for another month or more this time?"

He headed for the couch and finally sat down. Kathy left for home, and the whole family crashed and fell asleep for five hours. It was six thirty when I finally woke up. Holy shit! We slept the whole afternoon! Thank God for that big bowl of soup. I just reheated it, and that's what we had for dinner that night.

CHAPTER TWENTY-THREE

Mike and I have a very active sex life, but these past two months had been anything but. Mike is an anytime, anywhere type of guy, and after our five-hour nap, he was raring to go to say the least. But I told him that we shouldn't just yet. I mean he just came home from the hospital again after three days. I must admit I missed being intimate with him. I was glad that he was home again. I felt safe knowing that he would be sleeping next to me. I didn't want to be intimate just yet out of fear that Mike may hurt his back. But he did make a good point to me.

He said, "You know, we can't keep living in fear that I may get sick or hurt."

I said, "You know something, you're right, we can't."

Well as you can imagine we did have sex that night and you know what? It was good. It was like having sex with a new man. After our little romp in the hay, we snacked on some fruit, cheese, and crackers. Yup. Things were getting back to normal. Mike was becoming antsy at home and wanted to go back to work. I told him not to push himself and that when he felt he was ready, then he should go back, not before. He was worried that he was going to lose his job. I told him, "If they fire you over this, we would sue."

But Ben can be one of the biggest dicks to ever walk this planet, and I wouldn't put it past him to pull a dick move like that. Oh, he wouldn't do it right away; knowing this asshole, he would wait until Mike was back for a while and then do it. We made an appointment with the surgeon, Dr. Lopez, to see if Mike was well enough to be cleared to go back to work. His short-term disability was running out, and we really needed the income. I don't mean to sound selfish; as much as I didn't want Mike to go back to work, I knew he had to. Dr. Lopez did clear him to go back to work but with restrictions. Mike forced me to go back to work even though I didn't want to. I knew that we needed the income but still felt an enormous amount of guilt if I did. Reluctantly I did. Mike was not able to lift more than ten pounds, he wasn't able to climb ladders, and he wasn't able to push anything either. He also said that he wanted Mike to meet with his primary doctor as well to get clearance to go back to work.

So we made an appointment to see Dr. Chang. When we went to meet with him, as usual Mike was asked routine questions about his health. Mike then proceeded to tell him what happened to him in January. Dr. Chang nearly fell over. He just stood there and said, "Oh my god, how are you alive?"

Mike just said, "I was told I have a strong heart."

Dr. Chang looked at him and said, "I would say so. Speaking of hearts, I want you to see a cardiologist to see how your heart is doing."

Mike also told him that he was feeling a bit stuffed up. A bit stuffed up? That was an understatement! Did I mention how loud he snores! Good God, he could wake the dead! Dr. Chang examined him and said that he should see an ENT. Wow, this was too much! I thought to myself, *How many more doctors would he have to see? Would this be for the rest of his life?* I just didn't know.

Dr. Chang referred him to Dr. Lakshimi, who was an ENT, and Dr. Krish, who was a cardiologist. Dr. Chang told Mike that he was not going to clear him for work until he received all the tests results from both doctors. Do you have any idea how hard it is to get an appointment with a cardiologist? It took three weeks before we were able to see him! When we finally saw the cardiologist, he asked about Mike's health history and why he was referred to him.

When we told him what he had just been through, he said to Mike, "How the hell are you still alive? You should be dead!"

Mike just shrugged his shoulders and didn't know what to say except, "I have a strong heart." He really didn't know how close he had come to dying.

He wanted Mike to wear a heart monitor for thirty days to see how well his heart was functioning. We had to go to the downtown

Orlando office to get the heart monitor because it was a special kind of monitor he had to wear. He was given very specific directions on how to wear it. Well that sounds fun. He had to wear it while he slept too. Mike suggested that he wear it while we were having sex just to see what the monitor would show regarding his heart activity. Of course, Mike being Mike, he did. He wore it during our sexual activity. He also had to go for a stress test. And not just a regular stress test, it was a chemical stress test. Which means they combine an intravenous medication with an imaging technique (isotope imaging) to evaluate the heart.

The reason for this was because of his back. He was unable to run on the treadmill. So the medication that they had to inject him with put the same stress on his heart that running on a treadmill would. Well I'm guessing that by now you already know that Mike is not a big fan of needles. So getting him to do this stress test was not going to be easy. After the thirty days was up for Mike for the heart monitor, he had to go for the stress test. I took the day off to be with him. We got there early in the morning. He was in a panic because he knew that he had to have an IV. I kept trying to reassure him that everything was going to be okay. But Mike was a nervous nelly when it comes to needles.

Once they started the IV, I was asked to go back out to the waiting room until he was done. They did let me back in to see him in between tests because he wanted to see me. After the first round of tests, he was allowed a light snack. I knew that once he was done, he was going to be starving. I promised him that we would stop and get some food on the way home. That seemed to put him at ease a little. They then began the second and final round of tests. Once these were completed, we would be able to go home. Thank God. It was already a very long day; I could only imagine how Mike felt.

After all the tests were completed, we had to make a follow-up appointment to get the results. I was just hoping that this appointment wasn't going to be an all-day event like this was. When we arrived for the follow-up appointment, we checked in at the desk, and I was asked for a $35-co-pay. "*What!*" I looked at the girl and said, "His deductible has been met, there should be no co-pay!"

Mike put his hand on my shoulder and said, "Steady there, crazy lady."

I said, "*No*, I'm sick of everyone not doing their job properly! Instead of just assuming there is a co-pay, she should actually do her job and make sure there is none before asking for it!"

Mike looked apologetically at the girl and just shrugged his shoulders. The girl was a little shaken at my outburst and rechecked and said, "I am very sorry, there isn't any co-pay."

I made no apologies for my outburst and just gave her an "I told you so" look and sat down. We then met with the doctor, and he discussed the results with us. He told us that everything was normal with Mike's heart and that he was going to clear him to go back to work. He was going to forward the results to Dr. Chang as well. Both of us breathed a sigh of relief when we heard this. The only thing that Dr. Krish said was that he would have to take his heart medicine for the rest of his life. He told us that once you're on it, there is no coming off it.

Next I made an appointment with the ENT (ear, nose, and throat specialist), Dr. Lakshimi. Once we were at Dr. Lakshimi's office, the physician's assistant met with us. Again I was asked about Mike's health history. I once again told the PA about what happened to him in January. The look on the nurse's face was priceless when I told her everything. She looked at both of us in awe, like she couldn't believe what she was hearing. I thought she was speechless for a minute. Then it was like she was snapped back into reality, and she said was going to do a basic exam of his nose.

She did the exam of his nose and turned to us and asked, "When did he break his nose?" He looked at me with a puzzled look on his face. She asked him, "Have you ever broken your nose?"

Mike replied, "Not that I know of. It must've happened when I fell in the hospital."

She proceeded to tell us that he had a deviated septum as well. She told us that she was going to do a panoramic X-ray of his face. After the X-ray was done, we waited for the doctor to get the results. I saw the X-ray came up on the TV in the office we were in. It looked normal to me. But what the hell did I know, I'm not a doctor. Dr. Lakshimi came in and said that Mike's sinuses were completely clogged up, and it was wonder he could breathe. He wanted to schedule surgery to correct it. Oh great, more surgery. I was scared and nervous at the same time. After what happened with Mike's surgery back in January, I really didn't want him to have anymore. But I knew he needed it. Mike, surprisingly enough, wasn't that worried about it.

Dr. Lakshimi knew all about Mike's health history and assured me that he would take every precaution with this surgery. Reluctantly, I agreed to it. We still had to see the orthopedic doctor to see what was going on with Mike's back and why he was experiencing numbness on the right side of his head and his left leg. He was also having memory and speech problems. My head was spinning with all these doctors Mike had to see. Thank God for insurance because I would never be able to pay for all these procedures and doctor visits. The surgery was set for September.

The next doctor we met with was Dr. Evans, an orthopedic surgeon. He specializes in back surgery. With back surgery, the risks sometimes outweigh the benefits. One small mistake and Mike never walks again. In the back of my mind, I knew he needed it, but I didn't want him to have it. Dr. Evans did some basic tests on Mike in the office. He took an X-ray of Mike's back, and it was determined that Mike did in fact have a herniated disc and extreme weakness on the left side of his body, mainly his left leg. The weakness was so severe that he wanted to fit him with a leg brace, but Mike said no, that he was able to walk with a cane. But he didn't want to rush into surgery just yet because of what Mike had been through. The doctor instead wanted to try a different approach. He suggested that Mike receive some physical therapy as well as some pain-relieving shots. If after a few months this combination didn't work, then we would talk about surgery. The shots were to shrink the swelling of the disc and take the pressure off the sciatic nerve that was irritated.

The doctor that would be administering these shots was a colleague of Dr. Evans, his name was Dr. Ruben Myers. Hopefully it would work, but right now I was more concerned with Mike's nasal surgery that was coming up. Not only did they have to fix his deviated septum, they also had to remove all the polyps he had. We were told that due to him having a nasogastric tube while in the hospital, that's why he developed the polyps and the severe sinus problems he was having. Hopefully this surgery would work for his nose. If all these tests came back normal, Mike would finally be cleared to go back to work in late April.

CHAPTER TWENTY-FOUR

But before all this surgery was to take place, we wanted to take a trip back home to New York to see all our friends and family. We planned the trip for July. We booked the hotel on Staten Island where we could see everyone. I was able to get a great discount for the hotel through a program with my job. We were all excited about taking a road trip back home to New York. Oh, did I mention that we were driving? When the girls were little, we drove back and forth to Florida all the time. You may think we're crazy but we're not. Mike is not a big fan of flying, so we agreed that he would do the driving and that I would take care of the girls and prepare everyone's lunch. I thought that was a fair deal. But now that the girls are older, there was no reason for me to take care of them. So I shared the driving with Mike. All our friends and family were excited to see Mike after everything he had gone through. We had planned for our beagle to stay in the kennel while we were gone. While Mike was in the coma, his father and brother promised that they would buy him a new train engine. They even picked out of the engine that they would buy him.

Mike is an avid train collector and loved specialty engines. He has a massive collection that he only takes out on special occasions like Christmas. Mike was excited about going to the train store in Brooklyn, New York. The night before we were leaving, we were doing some last-minute packing when Mike's father called and asked if we were home.

Mike said, "Yeah, we'll be home. Why? What's up?"

His father said, "Not much, I have something to give you before you leave tomorrow morning."

Confused, Mike said, "Okay?"

Within fifteen minutes he was at our apartment. He didn't even come in; he just told Mike to come outside to his car. Mike went outside, and we stayed in the apartment and peeked out the window.

The girls were like, "What's Grandpa giving Dad?"

I said, "I have no idea. I just saw him hand an envelope to Dad." All I could see was Mike waving his hands and shaking his head no. At this point I was very confused and couldn't wait for him to come inside and see what was in the envelope. Finally he came inside.

We all asked at the same time, "What's in the envelope?" He opened it and counted out seven-hundred-dollar cash! My jaw dropped.

I asked, "What is the money for?"

He said to me, "Dad told me that he made me a promise when I was in the hospital and he keeps his promises. I told him no, that it wasn't necessary, that we had enough money, but he wouldn't take no for an answer. He just kept saying a promise is a promise. Go buy your train and enjoy your trip to NY. What was I supposed to do?"

I said, "Wow. Now we have more than enough money for NY! That $700.00 will be for your train and anything extra that we might need."

Now we were even more excited for this trip. Mike looked at me and said, "Yeah, now we can get more stuff at Novellis for the car ride home!"

Novellis is a local deli in Staten Island that has awesome food. Mike would walk there every Sunday morning with the girls to get cookies, cold cuts, and other stuff. He always got the girls gingerbread men cookies. They weren't really gingerbread, they were shaped like gingerbread men and had chocolate in the middle. The girls loved them. We were so excited that it was hard for us to sleep that night.

We left at six the next morning for New York. All Mike talked about was going to Train World and buying his engine. So off to New York we went. We met with family and friends and enjoyed our week. Mike did in fact buy his engine. The nasal surgery was set for September 16. It was going to be an outpatient procedure, which means he'll be able to go home the same day and recover from the comfort of his own bed. That was a little relieving to hear. Mike surprisingly wasn't as nervous as I was. Then again he wasn't the same person he was before. He came so close to dying and he was given a second chance at life and he was not about to turn back now. He told me that while he was in the coma, Saint Michael had come to him and told him that it wasn't his time and that he needed to come back to us and that he still had things to do. Now we are not religious people by any means, but this, this was a powerful message. Little did we know how true this was. We wouldn't know that for another year and a half.

Anyway, the day came for Mike's surgery, and, of course, I was nervous as all hell. But Mike, well he was cool as a cucumber. We arrived at the surgery center at 7:00 a.m. and waited. The surgery was going to last around two to three hours, and then we would be able to go home. I just wanted it over and done with. Honestly, I didn't want him to have any more surgery, but I knew that his back was next. While waiting his anxiety started to take over him, and he wouldn't go anywhere without me. I had to keep reassuring him that he would be okay. They came out and got us and led us back to the pre-op area. I was told to wait in the waiting room while they prepped Mike; once he was all done, they would come and get me. It wasn't long before they came to get me. I sat with him as long as I could until they kicked me out.

After two to three hours the nurses came to get me. First I spoke to Dr. Lakshimi, and he informed that what he took out of Mike's nose was the same consistency as that of peanut butter. He also removed a good number of polyps and that this surgery would become routine for Mike.

I asked him, "How often are we talking about?"

Dr. Lakshimi told me, "At least two to three times a year, and each time, it will get better."

A short time later, the nurse came out to get me. As I made my way back, I noticed that all the curtains where the patients were, were open except Mike's. I asked the nurse who was with me why his was closed and everyone's was opened. She didn't seem to have an answer. I took a deep breath and braced myself for what I was about to see. I pulled the curtain back, and I immediately went into panic mode.

There was Mike with and ice pack covering his eyes and what looked to be like an intubation tube. *Oh shit*, I thought to myself. What the hell happened now?

I slowly raised my arm and pointed to it and asked the nurse, "What is that?"

She said, "Oh, that's just oxygen to help him breathe." She said it so nonchalantly, like I was supposed to know what it was. I asked her about the ice pack, and she said it was to prevent swelling.

As soon Mike heard my voice, he asked, "Is that my wife?"

The nurse said, "I think so."

He says to her, "Is her name Anne?"

Before she had a chance to ask me, I answered him and said, "Yes, it is."

She then went to check on other patients. I asked him how he was feeling. He said to me, "Give me my sunglasses."

I said, "For what? We are inside."

He said to me, "It's too bright in here, just put them on my face please."

I said, "You have an ice pack across your eyes, where would you like me to put them?"

He said, "Just give them to me."

So I took them out of my pocketbook and handed them to him. He took them and put them right over the ice pack. "Aah, that's better."

I just shook my head and laughed. Suddenly he started saying out loud, "I have to pee. I have to pee."

I said, "Okay, okay, the whole recovery room doesn't have to know. Jeez, keep your voice down."

At that point the nurse peeked her head around the curtain and said, "Oh, does he have to pee?" I laughed and said yes. She said, "Okay, I'll go get him a urinal."

While waiting for the nurse to bring the urinal, the woman next to him was having a panic attack and sounded like she was going to throw up. The nurse came in with the urinal and stopped dead in her tracks and took one look at Mike and said, "Now who did that?" She was referring to his sunglasses being across his ice pack.

I said, "He did it. He said it was too bright in here."

She just shook her head and laughed. She handed me the urinal. I started to help him pee, and I guess I was not quite doing it right because he started yelling really loud and said, "I'm peeing on myself! I'm peeing on myself! Hold it down!"

Well the entire recovery room heard him. I was so embarrassed. The nurse was laughing and said to me that it was okay. Then he heard the woman next to him and said, "Oh great, now I have to hear this shit. Just what I want to hear is someone puking."

I looked at him and said, "Would you shut up! Everyone can hear you!"

He said, "I don't care who hears me. Can I go home yet?"

I said to him, "We're still waiting on the discharge papers."

He said, "Well what's taking so long?"

I said "I don't know. Just relax."

The nurse came in and said she had his discharge papers. She went over all the at home instructions with me and then had me sign off on the discharge papers.

Finally we were able to go home.

CHAPTER TWENTY-FIVE

When we finally got home, I was very relieved. I helped Mike get into bed. He wanted to listen to some music and watch TV. I put his headphones on him. I had to prop him up with our pillows because he had to sit upright the first twenty-four hours so blood wouldn't drip into the back of his throat. I went into the kitchen to fix myself some lunch because I was very hungry. After I ate, I went in to check on him. He was out like a light, so I turned the TV off as well as his music.

He woke up a little while later and said, "Hey, who's the bitch that shut my music and TV off?"

I said, "I am. You were out like a light."

Then he said to me, "Are you going to stay with me until Dad gets here?"

My jaw dropped. It took me a minute to respond, but I said, "You still think you're in the hospital, don't you?"

He said, "Yeah, so are you going to stay with me?"

I said to him, "You know you're home, right?"

He said, "No, I'm not."

I said to him, "Yes, you are!"

He said, "I am? Oh, I didn't know that."

I couldn't believe that he was remembering himself being in the hospital. After that he was like a jack-in-the-box. The man wouldn't sit still for five minutes! Every time I would put him in bed, he would get right back up again. It was unbelievable! At one point he got, up took my daughter Alex's arm, and said, "Let's go for a walk."

He must've walked around our apartment ten times. It was unbelievable! I told him that he needed to rest. I said, "I'm putting you back in bed, now don't move!"

He was like a child; he said, "But I don't wanna go to bed."

I said, "Too bad. I have things to do around the house and I can't if you're going to be up and down like a jack-in-the-box." I went back out into the kitchen and started to prepare dinner. Mike was going to have soup, and I was going to make hamburgers for the girls and myself. I had some housework to catch up on as well. I was hoping that Mike would sleep for a while.

But Mike being Mike, there was no keeping him down. If I could've strapped him down in bed like he was in the hospital, I would've. We had dinner. He did sleep for a while, but at 10:00 p.m. he was at it again. Disoriented, still believing he was in the hospital, I had to continually reassure him that he was home. He started roaming the house, and at one point he wanted to go outside for a walk. I had to physically restrain him and put him back in bed! I wondered if I would get any sleep at all that night. He kept referring to the gauze pad under his nose as "Stalin." I guess because he thought he looked like Stalin. Every time he needed it changed, he would say to me, "My Stalin needs changing." I must've changed it three to four times that night because he thought he kept bleeding through when he wasn't. Boy, I couldn't wait for the packing to be removed.

The next morning, we were to be at Dr. Lakshimi's office at 8:00 a.m. so the packing could be removed. The doctor also had to check on the stints that were put it in to make sure everything was doing well. This was going to be a very painful procedure when the stints were going to be removed. But for now just the packing was going to be removed. After the doctor removed the packing and checked the stints, he laid out a very rigid routine for Mike to follow for the next three weeks until the stints were removed. He had to flush his nose three times a day with a saline solution as well as use an ointment on the outside of his nostrils so they wouldn't become dry. He also wasn't allowed to blow his nose, and he wasn't allowed to bend over or lift more than 5 lbs. Even though Mike was a manager at the Star Palace Hotel, he still had to do manual labor. So explaining this to his manager, Ben Whitman, was not something he was looking forward to because Mike had absolutely zero support at work. Which pissed me off to no end. Dr. Lakshimi also gave Mike more medication to help keep any infection away that may occur. Mike remarked that he was taking more drugs now than he ever did as a teenager. Not that he was a big drug user. He may have smoked a joint or two but that was it.

Three weeks later we were at Dr. Lakshimi's office to have the stints removed. Mike described this as the equivalent to nails on a chalkboard when the doctor dragged them out of his nose. That's how painful this procedure is. The stuff that he took out of his nose was unreal. I've never seen so much mucus come out of one man's nose. For now this was then end of Mike's nasal surgery.

Mike was still receiving shots for his back and physical therapy. We still had to figure out what was causing all the numbness he was experiencing. So we made an appointment with a neurosurgeon, Dr. Cael. The doctor was going to perform a series of tests in his office as well as send Mike for a CT scan of his brain. But before all of that, he had to know Mike's health history and why we thought something was wrong. So once again we told the doctor what had been through, and he just couldn't believe that Mike survived all that. He just sat there with a shocked looked on his face.

Now came the tests. They were a series of electric shocks to the areas of numbness which would increase until Mike was able to feel it. Once we had the results of all the tests, we would know the reason for Mike's numbness. A few weeks later, the doctor called and asked us to come into the office so he would be able to discuss the results of all the testing that was done. We were so nervous because we didn't know what to expect. As it turned out, Mike did have some nerve damage from the lack of oxygen while he was in the coma. The doctor told us that it would take time for these damaged nerves to heal, or they wouldn't heal at all. So needless to say Mike still suffers from the numbness and occasional pain in his feet to this day.

After two to three months of Mike receiving these injections in his lower lumbar spine along with physical therapy, he didn't seem to be improving. It would help for three weeks and then the pain would return. So we scheduled another office visit with Dr. Evans, and it was then decided that Mike would need to have what is called a diskectomy, which basically is the removal of the disc that is pressing on his nerve. After the surgery he would have to go for more physical therapy to strengthen his leg.

Since Mike's nasal surgery had gone very well, he wasn't as nervous about his upcoming back surgery as I was. I called my daughter, Danielle, in New York and asked if she was willing to come down to be with me for Mike's back surgery. I told her that the surgery was set for the week after Thanksgiving on Thursday. She told me that she would come. That made me feel a little bit better. I needed Elizabeth to be home to take care of Alexandra as well as the dog. Wow, I was feeling overwhelmed with all of this. In the span of ten months, Mike will have had three surgeries! This was mind-blowing. I never thought he would've made it through what happened in January, let alone have two additional surgeries! He really is a walking miracle! I was praying that all would go smoothly with this surgery.

Danielle was flying down the day before. She was trying to cheer me up and said that she and I would go for coffee and breakfast while we waited for Mike. She knew that I loved doing that with her. When she and I worked together at Sam's Club, we would often get breakfast together. The girls were happy that she was here too. Like I said in the beginning, life is a little easier with her around. The night before the surgery, Mike had to take sponge bath of sorts. He was given a special wash to use to make sure that he had no bacteria on him.

The day of the surgery, we had to be at the surgery center by 6:00 a.m. so that they could prep Mike. The nurse came out to get Mike around 7:00 a.m. and brought him back to the surgical prep area. I was told that once he was ready, they would come out and get me so I can see him before the surgery. He had to take a sponge bath again with that same special wash he was given. I couldn't sit still. I was anxious to see him. The nurse came out a while later and asked me if I had Mike's inhaler. I asked her why she needed it. She said something like, "It's just a precaution."

She led me back to where he was, and when I saw him, it nearly took my breath away. He had two IVs going at the same time, and he looked very groggy. When I questioned the nurse as to why, she again said it was a precaution. I was seriously thinking about filing a lawsuit against County General. I felt they were responsible for everything that followed since Mike's surgery. The only problem with that though is proving medical malpractice. From what I was hearing, it was nearly impossible to prove, but I sure as hell was going to try. I mean as far as I was concerned, the hospital was at fault. But for now I just wanted Mike to get through this surgery.

CHAPTER TWENTY-SIX

While Danielle and I waited for Mike to come out of surgery, she went to get us some breakfast. I was starving, and I hadn't eaten anything at all that morning. I was too nervous to eat. I asked her to go to McDonald's and get me a bacon, egg, and cheese biscuit. Which is my favorite breakfast sandwich. While she was gone, I took out my iPad and started to play bingo on it. I needed something to take my mind off Mike's surgery. The waiting room was getting more and more crowded. I looked around and was amazed at how many people were there for surgery. My stomach was really starting to growl, and I was starting to wonder when Danielle was coming back. I was really lost in my game because I didn't hear Danielle come in the door. I jumped up to help her. Oh my god, the food smelled so good; I couldn't wait to eat.

Everyone was staring at us eat, but I didn't care I was so hungry. Then while we were eating, a nurse walked over to us and said, "I'm sorry, but you'll have to eat that outside of the waiting room. It's not fair to the patients who are waiting for surgery."

Well that was it; after everything that I had gone through with Mike, the last thing I needed was some nurse telling me where I can and can't eat. I looked up at her and I said, "I really don't care. I'm not going out there. I'm going to finish my food right here, and whoever doesn't like it, well that's just too bad." I think she was too shocked to respond. She just turned and walked away.

My daughter looked at me and said, "Mom, why would you say that? It's not that big of a deal, we'll just go out there and finish eating. Why do you always have to fight with everyone?"

I said, "Danielle, I'm halfway finished eating anyway, so who cares."

Danielle just shook her head and continued to eat her food. After we finished eating, we just sat there waiting for Mike to be done. I took out my iPad again and started playing Candy Crush this time. Danielle was so tired she curled up like a little ball on one of the chairs and went to sleep. Finally a nurse came out and said to me that Dr. Evans wanted to talk to me in private in one of the conference rooms. My pulse started to race. I was beginning to panic. I thought to myself, *Oh shit, what happened now. I can't go through this again.* I got up and went into the private conference room that the nurse directed me to and waited for Dr. Evans.

I sat down at the roundtable and was thinking the worst. Dr. Evans came in and sat down opposite me and proceeded to tell me that all went well with the surgery and that Mike should be able to go home soon. Oh, thank God. I was very relieved. He said that I would be able to see Mike soon. He informed me that he was in recovery now and that as soon as he was awake, I would be able to see him. I slumped back into the chair and breathe a huge sigh of relief. I thanked him for the information and headed back out to the waiting room.

As soon as Danielle saw me, she jumped up and came right over to me. She asked me, "So how did Dad's surgery go? Is he okay? When can we see him?"

I said to her, "Whoa, slow down. One question at a time. The surgery went well. He's in recovery, and we have to wait until he's awake before we can see him."

She said to me, "But he's okay, right?"

I said, "Yes, he's okay."

We both sat down and waited. The nurse came out a little while later and said that we were able to see him. She also said that Danielle should go get the car because Mike would be discharged soon. Danielle headed down to get the car. I gathered up my belongings and headed back to the recovery area.

I approached the recovery room filled with apprehension, not knowing what to expect. I noticed two nurses were sitting and monitoring Mikes vital signs. Of course, I hear Mike chatting away with the nurses. You would think he'd just shut up and relax. Nope not my husband. This man talks to anyone anywhere. When we reached the room Mike was in, the nurse turned to me and said, "Here he is."

I looked in and saw Mike lying peacefully in his bed. I didn't want to disturb him, but he must've heard me because he said, "Babe, is that you?"

"Yes, it's me. You're still pretty groggy from the anesthesia, so you shouldn't get up just yet."

He was like a child. "But I want to go home."

The nurse came back in and told us that Mike had to urinate first before he was able to go home. This was just a precaution to make sure all his organs were functioning properly after the anesthesia wore off. So, of course, Mike being Mike, he responded by saying, "Bring me a urinal, I can pee right now!"

The nurse looked at me and said, "I see someone really wants to go home. Okay, I'll be right back."

When she left, I helped Mike sit up and get out of bed. He seemed to be getting around rather well. I helped him get dressed too. I said to him, "Whoa, easy there. Don't push yourself. Okay?"

He looked at me and said, "Look, see I can walk. All I have to do is pee."

The nurse came back a few minutes later with urinal. She told us that once he peed in the urinal, it had to reach a certain line for him to be able to go home. I took it from the nurse and helped Mike try to pee. But it just wouldn't happen. I went to get some water for him to drink. After about five glasses of water, he tried again. But again, no success. The nurse came back and asked if he went. I said no not yet. She said, "Get him up and walking. That should help."

I looked at Mike and said. "Are you ready to go for a stroll, buddy?"

He stood up, held out his arm, and said to me, "Let's go!"

Little did Mike know that if he didn't pee, he wouldn't be going home. So I took his arm, and we started to walk around the recovery area. Mind you he was still hooked up to his IV pole. So there we are strolling with his IV pole around the recovery area. There was another man doing the same thing. Apparently this man had been walking around for a while, and he still couldn't pee. Mike had stopped and leaned against the wall so he could catch his breath. As we were standing there, we overheard the nurse talking to the other man and telling him that he was going to be admitted for the night and wouldn't be released until he was able to pee. Well that's all Mike had to hear. He looked at me and said, "Oh no, that's not happening to me. I will pee, and I will be going home. I don't care how many times I have to walk around."

We circled around at least three more times. By this time Mike said that he was feeling like he had to go. So we headed back to his room. He sat down on his bed to catch his breath. Then he stood up and tried to pee. Still nothing. So I went to get him more water to drink. He drank three more glasses. Again we went for another stroll around the recovery area. We passed the same gentleman along the way. Inside I was starting to worry why Mike wasn't having the urge to pee yet, but I didn't say anything just yet. After we circled around for the fourth time, Mike wanted to head back to his room and try to pee. We made our way back to his room, and I sat him on his bed so he could catch his breath again. Once he did, he stood up and tried to pee again. At last he was able to pee. But would it be enough? The nurse came back and looked at the amount of urine there was. She said it wasn't quite enough and that he needed to squeeze out a little bit more. Once again we went strolling. I thought to myself, *My god, hasn't he peed enough?*

This whole time that I was walking with Mike, Danielle was blowing up my phone with text messages, asking me when we were going to be done. She was waiting in the car for us and was getting anxious to go home. I told her, "As soon as Dad pees enough in the urinal, then we would be able to go home."

She let out this sigh and said, "Well tell him to hurry up. I'm hungry and want to eat."

I said to her, "You know you can't rush these things. He's doing the best he can."

After Mike and I went strolling for the fifth time, we headed back to his room to see if he was able to squeeze a little more out. I helped him sit on the bed and grabbed the urinal and held it for him so he could try and pee. Finally he peed in the urinal. I called the nurse and asked her to come look and see to see if it was enough.

She came in the room, and I held up the urinal for her and she looked at it and said, "Yup that's enough. I'll go get his discharge papers." Thank God.

Mike said, "I can go home now?"

I said, "Yes, we're just waiting for your discharge papers. Just relax, okay?"

Mike got all excited and said to me, "Help me get dressed. I wanna get out of here."

I looked at him and said, "Hey, take it easy, you still have your IV in your arm."

Mike said, "I don't care, I just want to go home. I'm sick of hospitals." I couldn't blame him. I texted Danielle and told her that we were just waiting for Mike's discharge papers and for his IV to be removed and then we would be coming down to the car.

The nurse came back in and said, "Okay, ready to get that IV out of your arm?"

Mike looked at her and excitedly said, "Let's do this."

So the nurse proceeded to take his IV out and Mike couldn't have been happier. After the IV was out, she went to go get his discharge papers. She read us the dos and don'ts that Mike should do, and since Mike was still heavily medicated, I had to sign the discharge papers for him. Without hesitation, I did so. He couldn't get in that wheelchair quick enough. I texted Danielle and told her that we were on our way down to the car.

She texted me back and said "Finally!"

She asked if we could stop for food on the way home. I said absolutely. I myself was very hungry. We got down to the car, and I let Mike sit in the front seat with Danielle. Of course, he wouldn't stop touching the radio dials. He was driving Danielle crazy!

She started to yell at him, "Dad, stop touching the radio! You're not driving, I am! So just lay back and go to sleep!" I told him the same thing.

"It's my car!" He yells.

I said to him, "You're acting like a child you know that? Just stop and let her drive, okay?" He finally sat back and closed his eyes. Danielle stopped at McDonald's and got some food for her and me as we headed home.

CHAPTER TWENTY-SEVEN

Once we were home, I helped Mike get into bed so he could rest and hopefully fall asleep. Danielle and I sat down and ate our food. I was very grateful that she was here. She was going to take the girls out bowling that night to spend some quality time with them. This year was a tough year so far; the girls and me had been through a lot with Mike being in the hospital as much as he was. Danielle's best friend, Michelle, was going out with them. The girls were very excited to go out with Danielle and spend time with her.

Since the Christmas tree was up, I decided to take a nice Christmas picture of the girls. This would be the first Christmas picture that I have of the three of them since Danielle moved back to New York. Like I said, in the beginning, they really looked up to her. They went out around eight. I must admit I was relieved that they were going out to have some fun. I was so tired, I just wanted to lay on the couch, relax, and watch TV. I felt like a big weight was lifted being that Mike's back surgery was over. I was hoping that he didn't have to endure anymore surgery. Three in one year was enough for me. He was going to be home for a day or two, and then he was going back to work. Even though he was a manager, he still had to do manual labor.

I said to him, "Isn't that what you have guys for? I mean can't you tell them what to do? You need to be careful and listen to the what the doctor says."

He looked at me and said, "I will. I will."

Mike did return to work two days later, and so far, things were going well. He was doing what the doctor said and letting the guys do all the heavy lifting for him. He was also going for physical therapy as well to help his left leg become stronger. He had to leave work early for some of his appointments, and at first they were okay with it, but then they started to give him a hard time over it.

Whenever he would tell Ben that he had an appointment, Ben would say, "You know you can't keep leaving early like this. It's getting out of hand."

Mike thought about it for a minute and then said, "Hey, wait a minute. Ray leaves early all the fucking time, and no one ever says anything about that. But me leaving early for appointments is becoming a problem? What the fuck, Ben?"

Ben just stood there and didn't say anything. Mike knew damn well that this was all coming from that prick Richard who was the new "dictator," not from Ben. Ben's a coward and didn't know how to stand up for his managers or his hourly employees. He was just a puppet, and Richard pulled the strings. Everyone knew that. He was a poor excuse for a chief engineer. Anyway Mike kept leaving early and didn't really care what anyone thought.

As I mentioned in the beginning, Mike was having terrible night terrors while sleeping. He would wake up in cold sweats and would scream about this or that. He was reliving what had happened to him in the hospital. I suggested that maybe he sees a therapist about this, but Mike is a proud man and said that these night terrors would pass. What could I do? He's a grown man, and I couldn't very well force him to go if he didn't want to go.

CHAPTER TWENTY-EIGHT

Things were going well for the next few months, but I had this uneasy feeling that 2017 was going to be another tough year, we just didn't know how tough it would be yet. Ben seemed to lighten up a bit about Mike leaving early for work for his doctor's appointment. Every now and then Ben would say something to him, but Mike always blew him off. Mike had made a full recovery and was back working full time. We were even planning another trip to New York in the summertime. Mike was even brave enough to get his first tattoo! It was a picture of me that he had taken, and he had it tattooed on his shoulder. Years of Mike being afraid of needles resulted in him getting this tattoo; because of what he had been through, he figured, *Shit, why should this be any different?*

He was still battling his night terrors but still refused to see a therapist about it. I figured that when he had enough with his night terrors, he would go and see a therapist.

In early June 2017, it had been a year and a half since everything had happened to Mike, and he was finally given full medical clearance from his team of doctors to resume full duties at work. And guess what? Richard couldn't have been happier. Why you ask? Because he was finally able to terminate Mike without the attachment of a possible lawsuit. Just when we thought things would be back to normal, the rug gets pulled out from underneath us. On June 17, 2017, at one in the afternoon, Ben and Richard called Mike into Ben's office and told Mike that due to his performance issues, they were letting him go.

Mike sat there, stunned and in disbelief. He stood up to hand in his keys and phone, and Ben rolled his chair back close to Richard, fearing that Mike might turn around and punch him in the face.

Mike was professional about it and said, "Here you go. Thank you and goodbye."

He was walked to his office like a fucking common criminal where he proceeded to pack his things and leave. While this was happening, I was at work and had no knowledge of this. Mike came home and called me at work to tell me what had just transpired. I nearly dropped the phone, and I just couldn't believe it. After hearing this, all these thoughts of how we were going to pay our bills were racing through my head once again. Then of course the anger was rising inside of me because I knew just how much of a kiss ass Ben is and how much of a prick Richard really is. Don't get me started on their HR department whom are just as phony. That prick Ben never called me once when Mike was in the hospital to see how Mike was doing or even to see if I needed anything. It just goes to show you the kind of people Mike worked with. Uncaring, untrustworthy phonies.

Mike proceeded to make several phone calls to his team to inform them of what really happened because he knew the truth would never be told. And of course, it wasn't. The men that he managed were told that Mike just decided to leave to pursue another opportunity. Which of course was a lie. It was then that we both realized how fake people can really be. I knew with all this happening that Mike's stress levels would be on the rise, and I again suggested that he see a therapist. This time he agreed. We found a great therapist named Katie. He started to see her once a week.

We also filed a workman's compensation lawsuit against the Star Palace for a slip-and-fall accident Mike had before he was medically cleared. Guess what? We won! He also was able to receive his unemployment benefits without any problems. We still planned on going to New York in July. We already had the money put aside for that vacation. The girls were going to the Outer Banks in North Carolina with Mike's father and brother, Tom, and Tom's son, Thomas, for a week, and we would be picking them up and continuing to New York. We had no idea what that summer would bring.

CHAPTER TWENTY-NINE

From what the girls were texting me, they were not having such a good time in North Carolina and couldn't wait for us to pick them up. I asked them what was going on. They told us that Mike's father and brother were fighting all the time and that was bringing them down. When I asked what the fighting was all about, they said that it was over how Tom disciplined Thomas. You see Tom, being divorced, was always trying to be the fun parent and let Thomas do what he wanted. Whenever Tom tried to discipline Thomas, Thomas would always try to push the boundaries. This was one of those times, and Mike's father interfered, and Tom lost it. So as a result they didn't speak the rest of the trip, which made the girls feel uncomfortable.

When we picked up the girls from Tom, Tom proceeded to tell us just how unpleasant the trip was. He described it as a vacation from hell. He said that he would never do it again, not because of our girls but because of Mike's dad. We went our separate ways. The trip to New York was just what we needed to get our minds off all the chaos of Mike losing his job. We reunited with an aunt of Mike's whom we hadn't seen in years. It was Kathy's sister, Margie, and her family. She has two sons, John and Ronnie, and her husband's name is Ronnie also. We had lunch with them at Applebee's on Staten Island. I had reconnected with Mike's cousin, John, on Facebook a few months before and kept in touch with him. Aunt Margie was like a little kid waiting for us to arrive. She was so excited to see us she started to cry.

We spent three hours eating and catching up. It was very nice. We also had plans to reunite with Mike's cousin, Teddy, on Tuesday in the city for dinner. Our plan was to go sightseeing for the afternoon and then head uptown and meet Teddy and his wife, Lori, for dinner. We visited the Freedom Tower because we had friends who died in the 9/11 attack. It was a beautiful and solemn sight to see. Mike's reaction to seeing the new transportation hub was that "It looks like a giant vagina!"

We looked for the names of our friends on the pools that surround the World Trade Center footprints and enjoyed some time in the park before heading uptown for dinner. We had an enjoyable steak dinner with Teddy, Lori, Danielle, and her friend, Nicole. Teddy, who is also a diabetic, is in and out of the hospital because he didn't take care of himself the right way.

On Friday we enjoyed our last night out with Mike's friends at a local bar named Joyce's Tavern. Before we knew it, the week was over, and we had to head back to Florida. The girls were going to stay an extra week with Danielle and fly back a week later. Our plan was to drive straight through on Saturday because we had to get the dog out of the kennel on Monday, and we wanted one full day of rest before we had to do that.

We left for home at 5:30 a.m. on Saturday morning. I had mapped our trip home on my phone, and it looked like it was going to be smooth sailing the whole way home. We made a rest stop in Maryland, and my map on my phone said that we should be arriving home by ten thirty that night. Well that wasn't the case because, of course, we hit traffic in Virginia and that delayed us 2.5 hours. Now I don't like driving on highways, which meant Mike was doing all the driving, and when it got dark, he was having trouble seeing. He described it as tunnel vision. I asked him if he wanted to stop, and he said no, that he just wanted to get home to his own bed and sleep. I agreed. We finally made it home at 1:30 a.m. We were so tired that we didn't even unpack the car. We just took in all the food we bought. We showered and went to bed.

We didn't get up until eleven thirty the next morning. We unpacked the car, and then we went to Publix to get some groceries. We were so tired that we didn't even want to cook. You know what we did? My mother had given us an Applebee's gift card for our anniversary, so we ordered take out and that was dinner. It felt like we were newlyweds again. It was fun. It was nice to have some time to ourselves without the kids or the dog. We had the whole week to be newlyweds again.

The girls came back a week later, and it was back to same routine again. Except that Mike wasn't working, which was fine. We were doing okay with the bills so far. He had withdrawn his 401k, which helped a lot. Oh, and remember that lawsuit I mentioned? Well we finally got the settlement which was ten thousand dollars. We also had his unemployment, which helped too. With Mike being home all the time, he was becoming bored. Not that he wasn't looking for a job because he was.

So one day he took me to work because he had an appointment with Katie, whose office was ten minutes from my job. Since I was early for my shift, I was sitting in the staff cafeteria just relaxing when my cell phone rang. I answered it, and it was Elizabeth; she said, "Mom, Dad's therapist just called and asked if he left for his appointment. I told them yes he did, but they said he isn't there yet."

I said, "Okay, well he probably hit some traffic and should be there soon. I'm going to call the office in a little while and see if he got there and then I'll call you."

She said, "Okay, Mom."

I waited about fifteen minutes and called the office. I told them who I was and asked the girl if Mike had gotten their yet. She said, "No, I'm sorry he hasn't arrived yet. If you would like, I can take your number and call you the minute he gets here."

I said, "Okay, here is my phone number. Please, call me the minute he gets there."

Now I was panic-stricken at this point. I thought, *Oh my god, what could have happened to him?* I kept looking at my phone, waiting for it to ring. I couldn't wait any longer, so I called the office back and the girl answered and said, "I was just about to call you, he got here a few minutes ago."

I breathed a huge sigh of relief and asked to speak to him, and she told me that he was with Katie. I asked her what happened. She told me that he said he got lost. Got lost? What? That doesn't make sense. I was a little alarmed when I heard that and would ask Mike about it when he picked me up. I called Elizabeth at home and told her that Mike finally got to the office. She asked me what happened, and I told her that he got lost. When Mike picked me up, I asked him how he got lost going to Katie's. He said that he had become disoriented and forgot where he was going.

I said to him, "Maybe we should make an appointment with the neurologist?"

He said, "No, I'm fine. I'm still getting used to going there."

I texted Danielle and told her, "Time to get Dad a cell phone."

She responded by saying, "What? Why?"

I told her that he got lost going to see Katie and I had no way of getting in contact with him and had to call the office. She said that she would look in to see how much adding an extra line to my plan was. Within a day Mike had a new cell phone.

A few weeks went by and Mike seemed to be fine. Things were back to normal, and we were dealing with Mike still being out of work in our own way. Nobody knew except Danielle, and that's how it would stay. It was the Monday before Labor Day, and Mike's brother called him and asked him for one hundred dollars. Odd but okay. Now with Mike still being out of work, we were certainly in no position to say yes, but we did anyway. He asked what the money was for, and Tom said that it was for some stomach medicine he needed. Mike told him to come for dinner that night and he would give it to him. He came for dinner that night, and Mike gave him the money with no problems. We laughed a lot and had a good time. Tom left sometime around seven thirty that night.

The next day Tom called Mike and thanked him again for the money. Tom always called him between four and five every afternoon as they would both be on their way home from work just to chitchat. Mike asked him how he was feeling, and Tom said that he was feeling great and that the medicine was really helping. Mike was happy to hear that.

On Wednesday Tom again called Mike and asked him what his plans were for Labor Day. Mike told him, "Not much because Anne has to work ten to six thirty on Labor Day. But don't worry I'll take Anne to work and then we'll come up to you and then I'll leave at six to pick her up."

Tom was happy about that. They discussed what they would cook. When the two of them cooked, it was always delicious, but they always made a mess. Mike said that he would talk to him more over the weekend to finalize the menu. Nothing could've prepared us for what was about to happen early the next morning.

CHAPTER THIRTY

On Thursday morning, August 31, 2017, at five forty-five, the phone rang. We both jumped up because we couldn't imagine who could be calling us this early. Mike picked up the phone and said, "Yeah, hello?"

All I heard was Kathy screaming, and I mean screaming hysterically. "He's dead! Tom is dead! He's dead!"

Mike was like, "Mom, what are you talking about?"

Again she screamed, "He's dead! Tom is dead! He's dead!"

I was frozen out of sheer shock. Next thing my girls came running out of their rooms because they hear Mike saying, "Mom, what do you mean Tom is dead? What are you talking about?"

Again she said, "He's dead! They told me he's dead!"

Mike looked at me and said, "Here take this. I have to go pee before it comes down my leg."

There I am standing there in shock, holding the phone and speechless because I couldn't believe what I was hearing. The girls came right over to me, and I just said, "Well I guess I'm not going to work today."

Mike came out of the bathroom and said, "I need to call Dad." He called his father's house and got his stepbrother, Jay, on the phone and said, "Jay, where's Daddy?"

Jay said, "He's in Puerto Rico."

I said to Mike, "Let me call your mother back and see if the EMTs are still there and talk to them before you call your father." I called Kathy back and asked her if the paramedics were still there, and she said yes. I said to her to let me speak to them.

She handed the phone to one of them and said, "It's my daughter-in-law."

The paramedic got on the phone, and I told him who I was and my relationship to Tom and asked if this was true. He said, "Yes, ma'am, he's been down for some time. He's passed away."

I asked him, "How did this happen?"

He said, "I don't know, ma'am, the coroner is on their way."

After I hung up with the paramedic, Mike called his father and told him the grim news about Tom. Now at this point Tom and his father hadn't spoken since the Outer Banks trip. So you can imagine his reaction. He dropped his phone, and all Mike heard was him saying, "My son, my son. Oh my god, how did this happen?"

Suzy then took the phone and asked to speak to me. Mike handed the phone to me and said, "Suzy wants to talk to you."

"Me? Why?"

Mike said, "I don't know."

I got on the phone, and the first thing out of Suzy's mouth in her broken Spanish-English accent was, "Annie, no bullshitting around. Is this true?"

I said to her, "Suzy, why the fuck would I make something like that up? I spoke to the paramedic myself, and he said yes, that Tom passed away." I couldn't believe that she thought I made that shit up.

She was like, "Okay, okay, I just wanted to make sure."

Can you imagine after everything Mike had been through over the last year and a half, he now has to bury his brother who was only forty-five! As we were driving up to Kathy's house, we were continually trying to contact my daughter Danielle who lives in New York; while doing this, Tom's ex-wife, Angela, called my phone. She told me that when Kathy told her what happened, she dropped the phone and screamed. I don't really believe that because she is a bitch. But I'll leave that for the next story.

We finally reached Danielle and told her the sad news. Pete, her boyfriend, thought Mike died judging from her reaction. She was having a panic attack and hyperventilating. Mike was telling her that she needed to calm down before she wound up in the hospital, and that was last thing we needed right now. She managed to compose herself and expressed how sad she was for Mike. She told him that she and Pete would be on a flight later that day.

When we arrived at Kathy's house, we saw two cop cars in front of the house. We entered the house, and Kathy was sitting at the dining room table, and as soon as she saw us, she came right over to us and just started bawling. She took Mike by the hand and showed him where Tom was.

She said, "Look, this is where I found him."

To be honest it looked like Tom was sleeping. I couldn't even look at him. I was so freaked out. I mean I watch a lot of criminal shows on TV and they show dead bodies, but to see it in person was a whole other thing. Mike was beside himself when he saw Tom's body. It's his only sibling. But he had to keep his composure for his mom's sake. He kept asking when the coroner was going to arrive, and they told him that he or she were on their way.

The past two years have been nothing but an emotional roller coaster for the entire Papsodero family. Let's just say that nothing surrounding Tom's death made sense. That's another story for another time.

CHAPTER THIRTY-ONE

After everything Mike has gone through, he is doing much better health-wise. He now has a much better job with Casino Resorts as chief of facilities, where he has zero stress and has a director that supports any, and all decisions that he makes. After the death of his brother, his PTSD became even worse. He continues to see Katie on a regular basis. He also has had two more nasal surgeries that were a success. The back surgery that he had has been successful. Mike is a different person as a result of his near-death experience and his brother's death. His new motto is "Life is short enjoy it." He tries to live his life to the fullest. He's always looking to try new things. He misses his brother terribly but remembers all the good times and family vacations they had as children and adults. Unfortunately, we will never really know the true cause of his brother's death.

As I mentioned before, we did try to sue but every lawyer we spoke with informed us that the cost of filing a lawsuit would out-weigh, what I could potentially receive. After speaking with many lawyers, I'm now convinced that they are nothing but ambulance chasers. Especially in Florida. That's all they advertise on TV.

As a final piece of advice, I would like to say that you should always get a second opinion before any kind of surgery. I was very fortunate that Mike made a full recovery. Someone else may not have. And as always you should keep the faith. I did.

ABOUT THE AUTHOR

Anne was born and raised in Brooklyn, New York. She married Mike in 1993. She is the mother of three girls, ages twenty-four, twenty-one, and fifteen. She currently resides in Orlando, Florida. She works full time for a major furniture company. She enjoys reading and writing and spending time with her family. This is her first time writing a book. Anne is now looking forward to becoming a full-time writer.